Pocket Picture Guides

Diagnostic Angiography

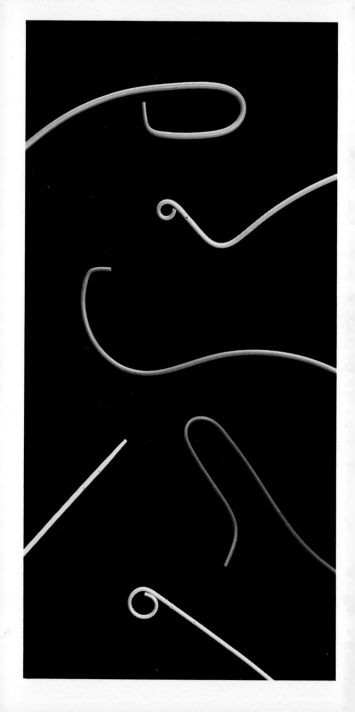

Pocket Picture Guides

Diagnostic Angiography

Robert J. Rosen MD

Director,
Vascular Interventional Radiology
New York University Medical Center
New York, USA

Gower Medical Publishing · New York · London · 1986

ISBN: 0-912143-11-8

Library of Congress Cataloging-in-Publication Data:
Rosen, Robert J. (Robert Jay), 1951–
    Diagnostic angiography.
    (Pocket picture guides)
    Bibliography: p.
    Includes index.
1. Angiography—Atlases.   2. Blood-vessels—Radiography—
Atlases.   3. Blood-vessels—Diseases—Diagnosis—Atlases
I. Title.   II. Series.   [DNLM: 1. Angiography—atlases.
WG 17 R813d]
RC691.6.A53R67   1986   616.1′3′0757   **86-22786**

Project Editor: Marion Geller

Design: Louise Bond

Illustration: Lynda Payne

Printed in Hong Kong by Imago Publishing Ltd.

Contents

Introduction

Angiography, like surgery, is a craft that cannot be learned from a textbook. This small volume is therefore not intended to teach angiographic technique, but rather to provide a brief atlas of common angiographic findings in various disease processes. The size of this volume dictates that only the more important or common processes may be covered. We feel that this compact atlas will be useful as an introduction or quick reference source for medical students, radiologic technologists, radiology residents beginning their angiographic training, or for radiologists in practice who could use a refresher in this specialized area.

The role of angiography has changed considerably in recent years. The introduction of computed tomography (CT) and ultrasonography several years ago was initially thought to signal the beginning of the end of angiography as a distinct discipline. Actually, advances in vascular surgical reconstruction, angiographic equipment, digital imaging, and, most of all, the explosive growth of interventional radiology have all combined to make angiography one of the most rapidly developing and exciting specialties in medicine today. Indeed, the number of angiographic procedures performed in most institutions, after an initial drop in the mid 1970s, has increased sharply in recent years.

There is no doubt that diagnostic angiography now plays a secondary role to CT and ultrasound in the diagnosis of abdominal diseases. Angiography is used in this setting primarily to classify or confirm certain diagnoses, to demonstrate the vascularity of some lesions, and to provide the surgeon with a vascular 'road map' prior to some operative procedures.

The diagnostic arteriogram is still the key study in the evaluation of patients with primary vascular disease. The incidence of atherosclerosis in our society means that a large number of examinations are performed in any institution with a busy vascular surgery service. Noninvasive studies can suggest the presence of impaired circulation, but only high quality angiography can provide the exquisitely detailed anatomic information that is required for making rational therapeutic decisions. The introduction of digital image enhancement as well as newer (nonionic) contrast agents promises to make these examinations less stressful than in the past. Many arteriographic studies can be performed now on an outpatient basis with almost no discomfort involved.

1
General Angiographic Techniques

Catheter Placement (Fig. 1.1)

Over the past 30 years various techniques have been employed to examine blood vessels radiographically. The most widely accepted method involves the placement of small catheters directly into the arterial system under fluoroscopic guidance. Catheter placement is performed using a technique described in 1953 by Seldinger: the artery is punctured percutaneously; a flexible wire, known as a guidewire, is passed through the needle into the vessel; the needle is removed, and a catheter is threaded into the vessel over the wire. Since the guidewire maintains access to the vessel, various catheters can be inserted or exchanged for one another through the same entry site.

Entry Sites (Fig. 1.2)

Certain anatomic locations are favored for access to the vascular system due to their percutaneous accessibility (a palpable pulse is required), their size, and their capability of being compressed directly to seal the opening after catheter removal. The most common entry sites are the femoral, brachial, and axillary arteries. The femoral artery approach is the most frequently employed, as it is quite safe and provides fairly direct access to most parts of the vascular system. Venous studies, of course, require direct entry into the corresponding veins.

Catheter Selection (Figs. 1.3, 1.4)

Once the vascular system has been entered, the selection of a catheter and its positioning depend on the structures to be examined. Although there are many variations, the two main categories of angiographic catheters are *flush* and *selective*.

Flush catheters, which may be straight or have a preformed "pigtail" tip, have numerous side-holes near the tip designed to deliver a large bolus into a major vessel, such as the aorta or pulmonary artery. Flush-catheter studies show more general anatomic territory, and provide less information about specific organs. Selective catheters, on the other hand, usually have only one opening, or end-hole, at the tip and are designed to be placed into smaller vessels for studies of specific organs. Of the many available shapes and sizes of selective catheters, some, such as the "cobra" curve, are useful for many selective studies, while others are designed to permit catheterization of a specific vessel, such as the gastroduodenal artery. These catheters are radiopaque, and are manipulated under fluoroscopic guidance. With experience, remarkably small distal vessels can be selectively catheterized.

CONTRAST INJECTION

When the catheter has been positioned, contrast is injected at a specific rate and volume, usually with an automatic injector. For flush studies contrast material is injected at a rapid rate whereas much lower rates of injection are required in selectively catheterized smaller vessels. Rapid sequential films are then taken. General guidelines for injection rates and filming sequences are available in angiographic texts, but these are often modified according to the specific situation at hand. Obtaining high-quality studies safely and routinely requires considerable experience.

COMPLICATIONS

By definition, angiography is an invasive procedure with certain inherent risks: those related to the contrast material, and those arising from the mechanics of insertion and manipulation of catheters within the blood vessels.

Contrast-related risks include allergy (ranging in severity from mild hives to anaphylaxis), renal toxicity, and neurotoxicity. Allergic reactions are not dose-related, whereas toxic effects to the kidneys and nervous system often are. Risks related to catheter insertion and manipulation include vessel occlusion, dissection (intimal injury), perforation, embolization, and hematoma formation at the entry site. Careful technique and experience can reduce but not completely eliminate the occurrence of these complications.

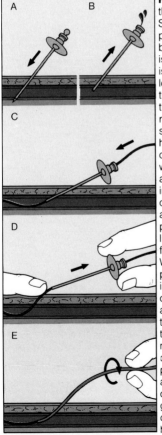

Fig. 1.1 This sequence shows the steps involved in the Seldinger technique for percutaneous catheterization of blood vessels. **A** After the pulse is located by palpation, the skin is prepped and infiltrated with local anesthetic. The vessel is then punctured at a 45° angle through-and-through with a removable stylet needle. **B** The stylet is removed, leaving the hollow outer cannula. The cannula is then gradually withdrawn until a strong spurt of arterial blood indicates intraluminal position. **C** The cannula is tilted to a shallower angle and a soft guidewire is passed through it into the vessel lumen. No resistance should be felt to the passage of the wire. **D** While the guidewire is held in place and manual compression is applied to the entry site, the cannula is withdrawn. **E** The angiographic catheter is then threaded over the guidewire into the vessel, generally with a rotary motion to ease entry. A short dilating catheter is often used prior to insertion of the angiographic catheter. Once the catheter is in the vessel, the guidewire is removed and the catheter is flushed with heparinized saline.

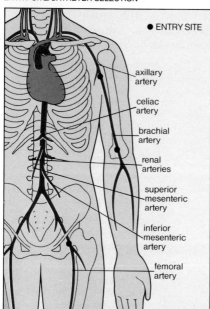

Fig. 1.2 The common entry sites used for angiographic examination.

● ENTRY SITE

axillary artery

celiac artery

brachial artery

renal arteries

superior mesenteric artery

inferior mesenteric artery

femoral artery

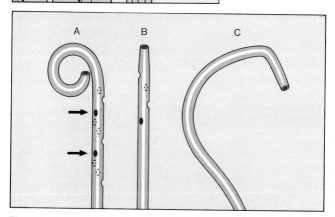

Fig. 1.3 Commonly used angiographic catheters. **A** The pigtail catheter is used for high-volume flush studies in large vessels such as the aorta and the pulmonary artery. The pigtail curve is an atraumatic shape that forces most of the contrast to exit the multiple side-holes (*arrows*) for a uniform bolus. **B** Another common type of flush catheter is straight with an end-hole and multiple side-holes. The straight configuration and end-hole add some risk of vessel trauma from the jet effect at the tip. **C** A commonly used catheter for selective study of branch blood vessels, such as the celiac axis, superior mesenteric artery, and renal arteries, is referred to as a cobra curve; the only opening is at the catheter tip.

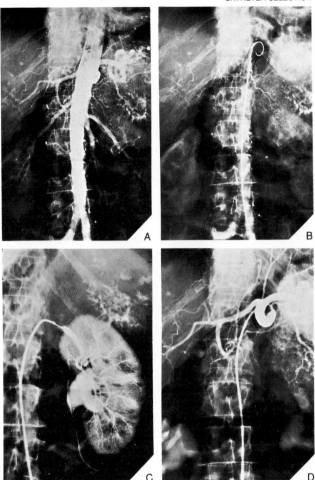

Fig. 1.4 Sequence of studies in the angiographic evaluation of a mass in the left upper quadrant. **A** Flush aortogram, performed with a pigtail catheter, shows filling of the aorta and its major abdominal trunks—celiac, SMA, renals, IMA. Some vessels are seen in the region of the calcified mass in the left upper abdomen. **B** A late-phase film from the same injection shows the calcification more clearly. Note also the normal bilateral nephrograms. **C** In a selective study of the left kidney, performed by inserting a cobra catheter into the left renal artery, the kidney appears normal and unrelated to the mass above it. **D** In a selective celiac axis study, also performed with a cobra catheter, the numerous pancreatic branches of the splenic artery that supply the hypervascular mass suggest that it originates from the pancreas. At surgery the mass was found to be a pancreatic cystadenoma.

2
Thorax

THORACIC AORTOGRAPHY

Thoracic aortography is performed by inserting a flush catheter, usually the pigtail type, into the root of the aorta by either the femoral, the brachial, or the axillary approach (see Fig. 1.2). Rapid injection and filming rates are required for optimal visualization due to the extremely high velocity of flow in this portion of the circulation. The best single projection for evaluating the entire thoracic aorta is the right posterior oblique (RPO) view. This projection throws the arch into profile, whereas on the anteroposterior view the ascending and descending segments of the arch are superimposed. In addition to the aorta itself, the study usually provides good visualization of the aortic valve and the proximal brachiocephalic vessels.

Thoracic aortography is most frequently indicated for evaluation of suspected aneurysms, aortic dissection, severe atherosclerosis, coarctation, trauma, and masses discovered on the standard chest film that are suspected of being vascular in nature.

The examination is generally quite safe. In addition to the risks of any angiogram, there is, however, the danger of neurologic injury, since the injection site is proximal to the origins of the brachiocephalic vessels.

Atherosclerotic Disease (Fig. 2.1)
Atherosclerosis commonly involves the thoracic aorta, but hemodynamically significant stenosis is extremely rare. The disease process may become clinically significant by involving the origins of the brachiocephalic vessels, with resultant neurologic sequelae or ischemic symptoms in the upper extremities. Ulcerated plaques may also serve as a nidus for embolization to almost any part of the circulation. Aneurysmal disease of the thoracic aorta (see below) is another common manifestation of atherosclerosis.

Aneurysmal Disease (Figs. 2.2–2.4)

Aneurysmal disease, which may involve any segment of the thoracic aorta, most commonly occurs in the ascending and descending segments, the transverse segment being relatively spared. Atherosclerotic aneurysms are by far the most frequent type, but other disorders may cause aneurysmal dilation or even rupture of the thoracic aorta. These less common causes should be suspected when there is selective involvement of the aortic root and ascending segment. Syphilis and connective tissue disorders such as Marfan's syndrome both result in degeneration of the media (cystic medial necrosis), which is the pathologic process underlying the dilation. When the aortic root becomes severely dilated, the valve may be affected, resulting in aortic insufficiency.

Atherosclerotic aneurysms are extremely variable in their appearance, ranging from long and fusiform to discrete and saccular. Calcification is often seen in the wall, and the margins of the lumen may show diffuse irregularity representing ulcerated plaques or a smooth featureless contour when laminated thrombus is present. Most of these aneurysms are asymptomatic and are discovered as a mass on routine chest films. When a patient presents with chest or back pain, leakage or impending rupture must be suspected and urgent evaluation and therapy carried out. Rupture of the aneurysm, associated with a high mortality rate, may occur into the pleural space, the mediastinum, or the pericardium.

Aortic Dissection (Fig. 2.5)

Aortic dissection, sometimes referred to as dissecting aneurysm, is a process involving disruption of the aortic intimal lining and dissection of blood between the layers of the vessel wall. Although the exact mechanism of dissection is not entirely understood, a primary degeneration of the vessel wall, commonly associated with significant systemic hypertension, is thought to be involved. Part of the nonsurgical management consists of decreasing the blood pressure.

Dissections may be localized or extend below the diaphragm as far distally as the femoral arteries. The major complications of this process are acute aortic valvular insufficiency, free rupture of the vessel wall, and shearing of branch vessels resulting in ischemia or infarction of almost any part of the body. The most common presenting symptom is pain: often sudden, severe tearing chest pain radiating to the back. In other cases ischemic complications, such as stroke, renal or intestinal infarction, or acute ischemia of the extremities may be seen. Therapy, usually involving surgery to repair the intimal, must be initiated rapidly, followed by measures to reduce the blood pressure.

The angiographic hallmarks of dissection are opacification of more than one parallel lumen and visualization of the intimal flap, which appears as a sharply outlined linear lucency within the contrast-filled lumen. In some cases catheterization by the femoral route is ruled out due to discontinuity of the lumen at this level with the "true" lumen of the thoracic aorta. A right axillary approach may be required in these cases to catheterize the aortic root. Thoracic dissections are commonly classified according to the anatomic segment involved: type 1 involves the entire thoracic aorta starting at the root; type 2 involves only the ascending segment; and type 3 begins just beyond the origin of the left subclavian artery and extends distally. The abdominal aorta is usually studied at the same time to determine the distal extent of the dissection process. Often a second intimal disruption, known as a re-entry flap, occurs distally where the false lumen has ruptured and again communicates with the true lumen.

Trauma (Figs. 2.6, 2.7)
Penetrating injuries that carry an extremely high mortality rate can involve any portion of the thoracic aorta. Angiographic visualization of extravasation is almost unheard of, since this would generally be associated with rapid cardiovascular collapse.

Blunt trauma tends to produce a specific type of injury to the thoracic aorta. The transverse segment of the aorta, just beyond the origin of the left subclavian artery in the region of the ligamentum arteriosum, is a common site of injury, usually involving a disruption of varying degrees of severity of the aortic wall. This type of injury is generally associated with chest trauma in motor vehicle accidents; fractures of the sternum and upper ribs are often seen in this type of injury. Complete transection of the aorta may occur, leading in many cases to almost immediate death; in some, however, the integrity of the adventitia, a very strong layer of the vessel wall, may prevent free hemorrhage and allow survival. An important clue to the presence of this injury, known as traumatic pseudoaneurysm or aortic transection, is widening of the upper mediastinal contour on the initial chest film. In a patient with a history of severe chest trauma, this finding indicates the need for emergency aortography, as the risk of delayed free rupture is extremely high in the period immediately following injury. In some patients the diagnosis of pseudoaneurysm, missed at the time of injury, may be picked up as a mass on a routine chest film many years later.

Thoracic Outlet Syndrome (Fig. 2.8)

The arteries, veins, and nerves of the upper extremity are subject to extrinsic compression at several specific anatomic sites. Typically, compression is associated with symptoms of pain, abnormal sensation, weakness, and occasionally atrophy or even frank ischemia of the extremity. This symptom complex is known as thoracic outlet syndrome. Clinical tests and maneuvers can be performed to elicit characteristic findings, such as positional loss of distal pulses, but arteriography or venography is often required to confirm the diagnosis prior to surgery.

Arterial compression may be evaluated on an aortic arch study or a selective subclavian arteriogram. The initial study is performed with the arm in neutral position, followed by repeat studies using various positions designed to demonstrate extrinsic compression by muscles, tendons, or bony structures.

Venous compression may also occur, with symptoms of arm swelling and venous engorgement; thrombosis may develop also as a result of the extrinsic compression. The veins are studied by simply injecting contrast through a vein in the hand or arm (see Chapter 5).

Pulmonary Angiography (Figs. 2.9–2.13)

Pulmonary angiography is performed by passing a catheter through the venous circulation and the right heart and into the pulmonary arteries where the contrast injection is made. Its most important application by far is in the diagnosis of pulmonary embolism. Other available studies, including radionuclide lung scanning, can suggest the diagnosis, but direct pulmonary angiography is universally considered the definitive study to confirm the diagnosis. Since many clinical conditions can mimic pulmonary embolism, and anticoagulation therapy carries significant risk, diagnostic specificity is extremely important.

Although contrast injection into the right atrium or the main pulmonary artery has been employed in performing this study, most angiographers now prefer more selective injections into the right or left pulmonary arteries. The radionuclide lung scan results serve as a guide to the areas of highest suspicion. Selective injections provide the highest-quality images, which are essential in finding small emboli in branch vessels. Oblique and magnification views may also be necessary to clarify questionable findings. The sine qua non of pulmonary embolus on an angiogram is visualization of a lucent filling defect within a contrast-filled vessel. Poor filling, cut-off vessels, and areas of apparently decreased perfusion are all nonspecific findings.

While pulmonary angiography involves certain risks, overemphasis of these risks can result in underutilization of an important diagnostic modality. Cardiac arrhythmias—particularly premature ventricular contractions—though common as the catheter is passed through the right side of the heart, are nearly always transient and generally require no specific therapy. Certain patients with irritable myocardium or preexisting heart blocks may be at increased risk. Acute right heart failure (cor pulmonale) is another risk, nearly always associated with severe preexisting pulmonary hypertension. For this reason, pulmonary arterial pressures are usually measured directly at the time of catheterization. If significant elevation is discovered, the injection rate and volume may be reduced or the study deferred.

Other indications for performing pulmonary arteriography include its occasional use in preoperative evaluation of tumor encasement in patients with neoplasms, an indication of non-resectability, as well as its use in demonstrating pulmonary arteriovenous malformations (AVM), which are uncommon except in patients with Rendu-Osler-Weber syndrome. In the latter case pulmonary AVM may be clinically significant for two reasons: (1) if large or multiple, they may markedly reduce systemic oxygenation and (2) they may result in paradoxical systemic embolism due to loss of the normal filter of the pulmonary capillary bed. Brain abscess is the most dangerous complication of this event. Transcatheter embolization using flow-guided detachable balloons provides an extremely effective nonsurgical alternative to surgical resection of the involved portion of lung.

Bronchial Arteriography (Fig. 2.14)

Selective angiography of the bronchial arteries, small systemic vessels that supply the lung parenchyma and tracheobronchial tree, is technically difficult. It is most often employed in patients with severe hemoptysis in whom all other studies, including bronchoscopy, have failed to clarify the site of bleeding. In addition to actual extravasation, the study may demonstrate areas of abnormal hypervascularity due to chronic inflammation, such as in severe tuberculosis and cystic fibrosis, or even arteriovenous malformation. Embolization may also be employed to control hemoptysis nonsurgically.

The main risk of bronchial angiography is neurologic injury related to inadvertent injection of the anterior spinal artery supplying the thoracic spinal cord. This vessel may originate from the bronchial artery trunk or from combined bronchial-intercostal trunks.

Superior Vena Cava (Fig. 2.15)

Venography of the superior vena cava (SVC) is most frequently indicated in the evaluation of suspected "superior vena cava syndrome." This symptom complex is associated with obstruction of the SVC and includes head, neck, and periorbital edema, venous distension, cyanosis, and, in some cases, syncope. By far the most common cause of obstruction is mediastinal tumor, which either invades or severely compresses the vein. This syndrome may also be seen with mediastinal fibrosis or massive mediastinal adenopathy of benign origin.

The SVC can be studied from an intravenous arm injection, which usually suffices if there is SVC obstruction. Typical findings include peripheral venous engorgement and filling of numerous collateral venous pathways in the neck and chest wall. These collaterals are seen in all but the most acute obstructions. If the SVC is patent or incompletely occluded, a peripheral venous injection produces poor opacification due to a large volume of unopacified blood inflow. Alternative methods of study include passing a catheter from the arm into the subclavian vein or SVC, as well as simultaneous contrast injection into both arms.

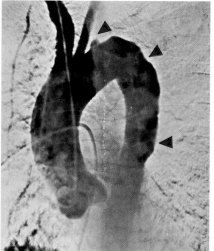

Fig. 2.1 Subtraction film in the RPO projection of the thoracic aorta in a 62-year-old man with symptoms of exertional pain in the left arm. Note the occlusion of the proximal left subclavian artery (*arrow* 1), as well as diffuse atherosclerotic disease of the transverse and descending thoracic aorta (*arrows* 2).

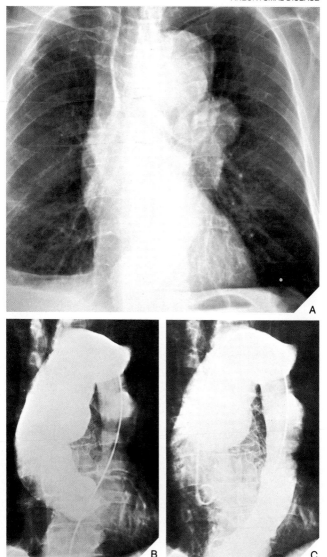

Fig. 2.2 A An 80-year-old man was found to have a mediastinal mass on routine examination that appeared related to the aortic shadow. **B, C** Thoracic aortograms in the AP projection show a long segment of severe aneurysmal disease involving the transverse and proximal descending aorta. **D** A repeat injection in the RPO projection demonstrates the anatomy more clearly, particularly the relationship of the aneurysm to the brachiocephalic vessels.

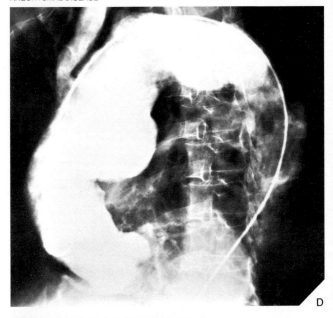

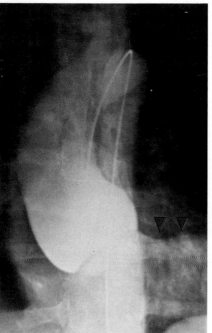

Fig. 2.3 A 53-year-old man with known Marfan's syndrome presented with decreasing exercise tolerance and a loud murmur of aortic insufficiency. Thoracic aortogram (AP view) demonstrates aneurysmal dilation of the aortic root and the ascending segment, typical of the aneurysmal disease seen in connective tissue disorders. The contrast-filled left ventricle (*arrows*) reflects severe incompetence of the aortic valve.

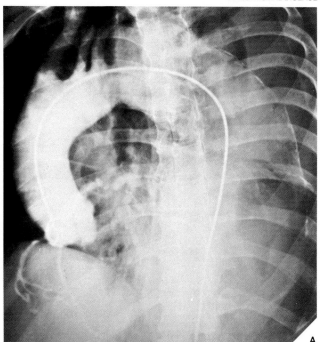

A

Fig. 2.4 A 72-year-old man presented in shock following an episode of severe "tearing" chest pain. On the plain chest film (not shown), the left hemithorax was completely opacified. **A, B** An emergency thoracic aortogram in the RPO projection demonstrates a huge descending thoracic aneurysm rupturing into the left chest. Curvilinear calcification is seen outlining the wall of this massive aneurysm. The patient died during attempted surgical repair.

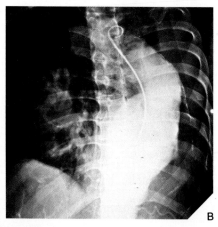

B

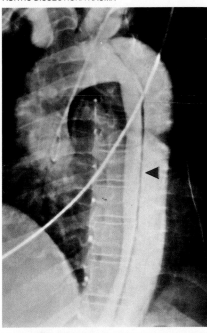

Fig. 2.5 A 33-year-old man with a longstanding history of severe hypertension was admitted with severe chest pain radiating to the back. Thoracic aortogram obtained via the axillary approach demonstrates the typical findings of a type 3 aortic dissection. The sharply outlined lucency (*arrow*) represents the intimal flap separating the true and false lumina.

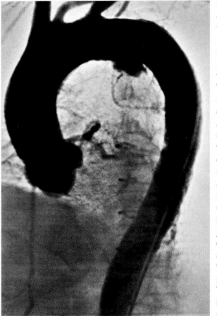

Fig. 2.6 A 58-year-old man was admitted with multiple injuries, including severe sternal trauma, sustained in a motor vehicle accident. Widening of the upper mediastinal contour noted on his admission chest film (not shown) indicated the need for emergency aortography. The aortogram in the RPO projection demonstrates a saccular outpouching just beyond the origin of the left subclavian artery—a finding typical of traumatic pseudoaneurysm. The intact adventitial layer prevented free rupture.

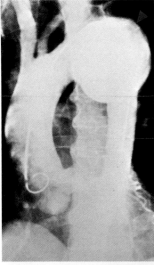

Fig. 2.7 In some patients the diagnosis of aortic transection is missed at the time of initial injury. The resulting chronic pseudoaneurysm (*arrow*) may be picked up as a mass on routine chest examination many years later. In this patient trauma occurred 20 years previously. Surgery is generally recommended, as delayed rupture is a constant threat.

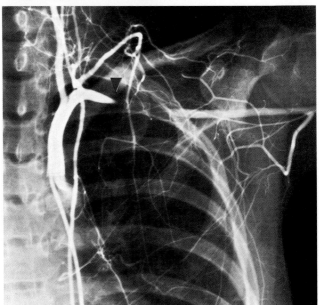

Fig. 2.8 A 15-year-old girl presented with complaints of abnormal sensation and weakness in the left hand, suggestive of thoracic outlet syndrome. A selective subclavian arteriogram (not shown), obtained with the arm in neutral position, showed no abnormalities. On abduction of the arm, extrinsic compression to the point of occlusion (*arrow*) of the subclavian artery becomes evident.

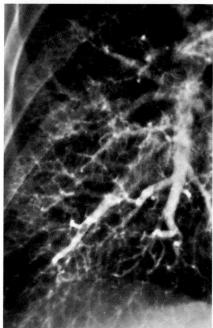

Fig. 2.9 Pulmonary angiography represents the "gold standard" in the diagnosis of pulmonary embolism. Findings can be quite subtle when the emboli are small and lodged in peripheral branches, but visualization of a lucent filling defect (*arrow*) within a contrast-filled pulmonary artery is diagnostic. In some cases oblique films or magnification views are required to make the diagnosis.

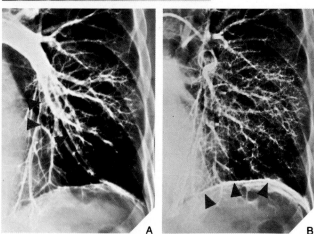

Fig. 2.10 A 29-year-old man presented with acute shortness of breath and severe left-sided pleuritic pain. Lung scan (not shown) demonstrated a perfusion defect at the left base, and the chest film (not shown) was within normal limits. **A** A selective left pulmonary arteriogram reveals several filling defects in lower lobe branch vessels (*arrows*). **B** A later-phase film shows marked pleural hyperemia at the lung base (*arrows*), an unusual finding.

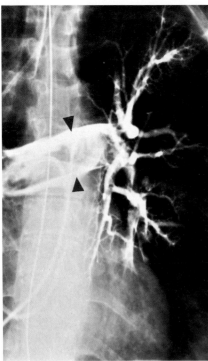

Fig. 2.11 Massive pulmonary embolism may result in shock or even sudden death. The only effective therapy for the most severe cases is emergency surgical embolectomy. This case represents a saddle embolus, demonstrated as a huge, lucent filling defect (*arrows*) in the main pulmonary artery, as well as in both right and left pulmonary arteries.

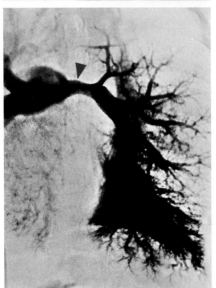

Fig. 2.12 A 58-year-old woman presented with symptoms of recurrent pulmonary embolism. A perfusion scan (not shown) revealed decreased flow to the left lung. The arteriogram shows narrowing of the proximal left main pulmonary artery (*arrow*). Eventually, the encasement was determined to be the result of a large central bronchogenic carcinoma.

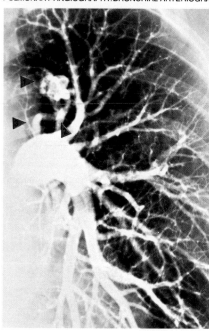

Fig. 2.13 A 48-year-old woman with known Rendu-Osler-Weber syndrome presented with increasing dyspnea on exertion and several lobulated parenchymal soft tissue densities on chest radiography (not shown). A left pulmonary arteriogram demonstrates an arteriovenous malformation in the upper lobe (*arrow* 1) fed by a pulmonary artery branch (*arrow* 2) and drained by a single pulmonary vein (*arrow* 3). It was successfully treated by selective embolization using a detachable balloon.

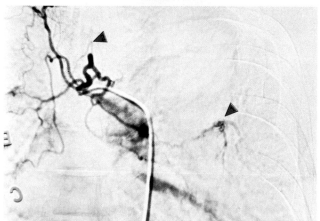

Fig. 2.14 A 37-year-old man presented with several episodes of massive hemoptysis. A selective injection of the bronchial trunk shows branches to the left and right lungs. Note the presence of a small arteriovenous fistula between the branches of a left bronchial artery and a pulmonary artery (*arrow* 1). Also note filling of the anterior spinal artery (*arrow* 2), which may share a common trunk with the bronchial circulation. The hairpin shape and midline position is characteristic of this critically important vessel.

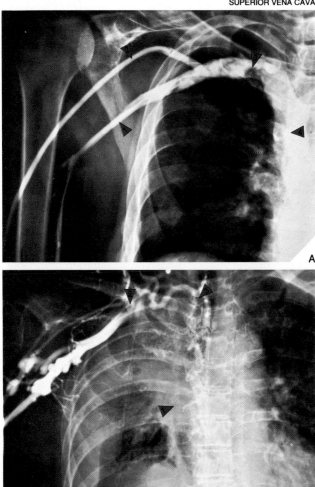

Fig. 2.15 **A** Study of right subclavian vein and superior vena cava from right antecubital vein contrast injection. Note normal filling of the basilic (*arrow 1*) and cephalic (*arrow 2*) veins, which then fill the subclavian vein (*arrow 3*) and finally the normal superior vena cava (*arrow 4*). The lucent defects within the contrast filled subclavian vein represent inflow of unopacified blood from venous tributaries. **B** A similar upper extremity venogram performed on a patient with superior vena cava syndrome due to a large bronchogenic carcinoma in the right lung (*arrow 1*). Note the complete obstruction of the subclavian vein (*arrow 2*) as well as filling of venous collaterals (*arrow 3*) bypassing the obstructed superior vena cava.

3
Nonselective Abdominal Studies

Aortography may be performed to evaluate abnormalities of the abdominal aorta itself (aneurysm, dissection), or as a general survey of the intra-abdominal organs. The study is performed by inserting a flush catheter into the abdominal aorta by one of three approaches: femoral, axillary, or translumbar.

Selective angiography is performed by inserting pre-shaped catheters into branches of the aorta under fluoroscopic guidance. Much more detailed images of individual abdominal organs are obtained with these selective contrast injections than with a simple flush aortogram.

DISORDERS OF THE ABDOMINAL AORTA

Aneurysmal Disease (Figs. 3.1, 3.2)

The diagnosis of abdominal aortic aneurysm is made generally by physical examination, and confirmed by ultrasound or CT. Angiography is used to provide a road map for the surgeon, showing the anatomic extent of the aneurysm, and its relationship to important branch vessels, particularly the renal arteries.

Occlusive Atherosclerotic Disease (Figs. 3.3–3.5)

Atherosclerosis of the abdominal aorta affects the infrarenal segment most commonly, with associated involvement of the iliac vessels. Findings range from localized plaques, which may ulcerate and embolize distally, to severe narrowing, or even complete occlusion. When it develops gradually, even complete occlusion of the infrarenal aorta or iliac vessels is remarkably well tolerated by most patients due to the enormous reserve of potential collateral circulation in the abdomen and pelvis. The Leriche syndrome is the clinical complex associated with aortic occlusion, which consists of buttock and thigh claudication, impotence in males, and absent femoral pulses.

Aortic Dissection (Fig. 3.6)
Aortic dissection is described in detail in Chapter 2. This disruption of the intima may be due to intrinsic disease of the vessel wall (atherosclerosis, medial necrosis, arteritis) or trauma (including iatrogenic). Most dissections begin in the thoracic aorta (see Fig. 2.5), but may extend to involve the abdominal aorta and its branches. The angiographic hallmarks of dissection are the "intimal flap," and the presence of more than one lumen.

Renal Vascular Disease (Figs. 3.7–3.10)
Renal angiography is frequently employed to investigate acute or chronic obstructions of the renal arterial circulation. Chronic obstruction of the main renal artery is commonly encountered in atherosclerosis. Plaques can severely narrow the vessel lumen at its origin or from the abdominal aorta, or there may be stenoses within the renal artery itself. The most common clinical presentation of this type of lesion is uncontrollable hypertension. If the occlusive disease is bilateral and severe enough, frank renal insufficiency may occur. Fibromuscular dysplasia is a distinctive lesion generally found in younger patients that also causes obstruction of renal arterial flow. It appears angiographically as a weblike stenosis, or a series of tight stenoses producing a "beaded" appearance. The lesion is often bilateral and may be encountered in blood vessels in other parts of the body of these same patients.

Acute renal artery occlusion is usually manifested clinically as renal infarction. The clinical symptoms include flank pain, nausea and vomiting, fever, and, in some cases, hematuria. Acute occlusion may be due to aortic dissection, embolic disease, or thrombosis of a previously stenotic artery.

Renal vein thrombosis is encountered in both children and adults. In children it is generally associated with severe dehydration and a poor prognosis. In adults there are numerous cases including generalized systemic disorders as well as renal inflammatory disease.

Acute renal vein occlusion may result in hemorrhagic infarction, while gradual renal vein thrombosis may be well tolerated if there is time for collateral drainage to develop. Renal vein thrombosis may be seen in association with the nephrotic syndrome. The renal venogram is diagnostic, demonstrating thrombus within the vein.

Pelvic Angiography (Figs. 3.11, 3.12)

Pelvic hemorrhage due to trauma, surgery, or tumor may be massive, and finding the source is notoriously difficult when attempted surgically. Pelvic angiography and selective embolization have proved lifesaving in many of these cases.

Arteriovenous malformations occur infrequently, but are found relatively commonly in the pelvis, generally supplied by branches of the hypogastric arteries as well as other pelvic vessels. These lesions tend to progress steadily, and have a marked tendency to recur after attempted surgical excision or ligation of feeding vessels. A complete angiographic evaluation to determine the extent of a lesion and the involvement of feeding vessels is mandatory prior to any attempted therapy. Recent advances in transcatheter embolization techniques, particularly the use of liquid agents, have allowed this to be used increasingly as a primary therapeutic modality with encouraging preliminary results.

Aside from investigating such specific vascular abnormalities, angiography is not often used in studying the pelvic organs.

Abdominal Venous Studies (Figs. 3.13, 3.14)

Leg venography usually allows visualization of the venous system up to the level of the iliac veins. In order to study the inferior vena cava, direct catheterization via a femoral vein puncture is required. Inferior vena cavography is performed in the evaluation of thromboembolic disease, to investigate unexplained lower extremity edema, and prior to surgery for large tumors that may be invading, compressing, or otherwise involving the inferior vena cava.

It is normal to see certain filling defects in the contrast-filled inferior vena cava, which represent inflow of unopacified blood from various tributary veins, including the iliac, renal, and, sometimes, the hepatic veins. Usually these filling defects appear to change in configuration from one film to the next in the angiographic series. Occasionally, it may be difficult to exclude a true filling defect, such as a blood clot, extension or tumor thrombus, from the renal vein orifice. In such cases, careful selective catheterization of the tributary vein in question may be required. It is important to keep in mind that the vena cava is a relatively slow-flow system, which may be markedly affected by changes in inspiration or intra-abdominal pressure.

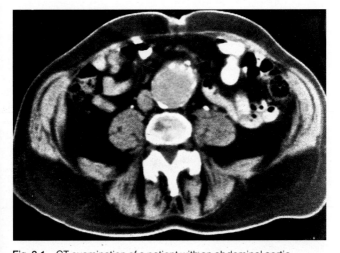

Fig. 3.1 CT examination of a patient with an abdominal aortic aneurysm demonstrates the contrast-filled lumen (*arrows*) as well as the laminated thrombus. Though this examination clearly demonstrates the relationship of the aorta to surrounding organs, the transverse orientation can be misleading at times, particularly when attempting to determine the relationship of the aneurysm to the renal arteries.

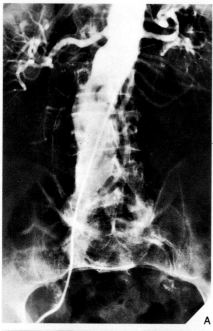

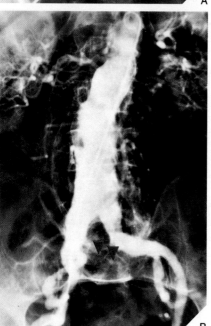

Fig. 3.2 **A** Abdominal aortogram of 79-year-old male who presented with a pulsatile abdominal mass. The catheter has been inserted from the femoral artery, and the injection made at the level of the renal arteries (*arrow* 1). Note the presence of a "neck" (*arrow* 2) between the renal artery origin and the beginning of the aneurysm. Also note the presence of a thin curvilinear calcification (*arrow* 3), which shows the true outer wall of the aneurysm. The space between this calcification and the lumen opacified by contrast represents mural thrombus. **B** As in most abdominal aortic aneurysms, the dilation extends into both common iliac arteries (*arrows*), while the external iliac arteries are of relatively normal caliber.

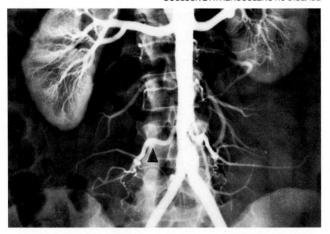

Fig. 3.3 Aortogram of a 44-year-old woman who presented complaining of claudication in both lower extremities, and was found to have absent femoral pulses bilaterally. The examination was performed therefore via an axillary approach. This midstream aortogram demonstrates a normal upper abdominal aorta and iliac segments, however, there is a large irregular plaque involving the left lateral aspect of the lower abdominal aorta (*arrow* 1). The hypertrophied lumbar arteries just above this level (*arrow* 2) confirm the hemodynamic significance of this lesion. This type of lesion often progresses to complete lower aortic occlusion, as is seen in Figure 3.5.

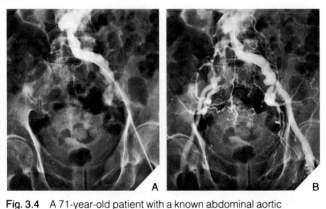

Fig. 3.4 A 71-year-old patient with a known abdominal aortic aneurysm, and an absent right femoral pulse. **A** This flush pelvic injection demonstrates aneurysmal disease of the lower abdominal aorta and the left common iliac artery. The right common iliac artery is completely occluded (*arrow*) at its origin from the aorta. **B** A slightly later phase film demonstrates prompt reconstitution of the external iliac artery (*arrow* 1) by the numerous collateral pathways, including the lumbar (*arrow* 2) and middle sacral arteries (*arrow* 3).

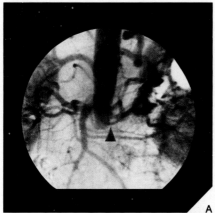

Fig. 3.5 A A 57-year-old man with the classic symptoms of Leriche syndrome (buttock and thigh claudication, impotence). Absent femoral pulses were noted on physical examination. A digital intravenous examination demonstrates complete occlusion of the abdominal aorta just below the level of the renal arterial origins (*arrow*). B, C These are demonstrations of the collateral reconstitution of both external iliac and common femoral arteries. This type of intravenous examination is considerably safer and far easier to perform than transaxillary or translumbar aortography in the evaluation of this type of occlusive disease.

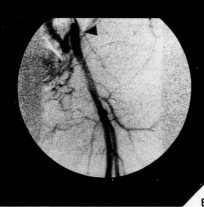

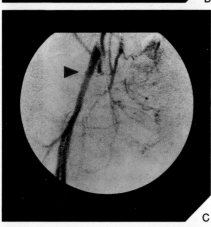

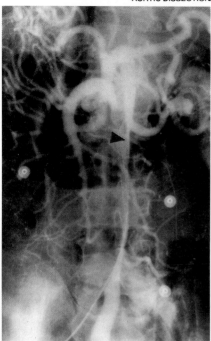

Fig. 3.6 A patient with a longstanding history of hypertension presented with abdominal and back pain of sudden onset. The aortogram demonstrates the bizarre appearance of the aortic lumen, which exhibits sharply tapered narrowing (*arrow*), and failure of filling of the right renal artery from the main lumen. This type of dissection usually originates in the thoracic aorta, and may result in disastrous clinical sequelae due to ischemia of any of the abdominal viscera.

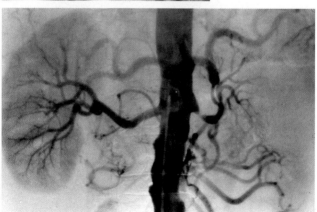

Fig. 3.7 A subtraction film from a flush aortogram that demonstrates a tight proximal stenosis of the left renal artery. The left kidney is considerably smaller than the right one due to longstanding impairment of blood flow. This type of lesion can be treated by bypass surgery or balloon angioplasty. If the kidney has been damaged too severely by chronic ischemia ("end stage"), nephrectomy may be the only treatment. The patient's clinical problem was uncontrollable hypertension.

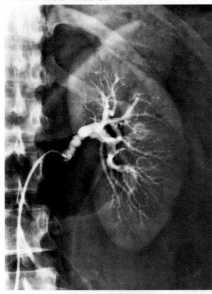

Fig. 3.8 A selective left renal arteriogram of a young woman with severe hypertension. The study demonstrates a series of band-like stenoses in the midportion of the main renal artery. This finding is characteristic of fibromuscular dysplasia. This type of lesion is encountered most often in young women, and is often bilateral.

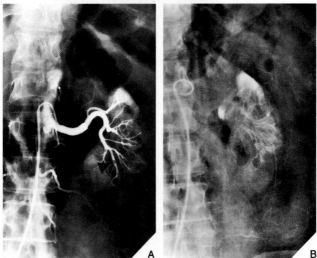

Fig. 3.9 **A** Small filling defects typical of emboli within intralobar branches of the renal artery are demonstrated on this selective left renal arteriogram of a 57-year-old woman. The patient presented with longstanding rheumatic mitral valvular disease, and the acute onset of left flank pain and microscopic hematuria. **B** The late-phase film shows a patchy nephrogram, with stasis in the embolized areas. Since the renal arterial separation is an "end circulation," acute arterial occlusions generally lead to infarction.

30

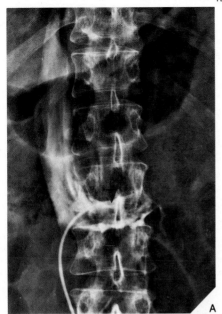

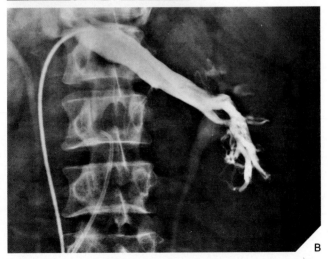

Fig. 3.10 **A** A selective left renal venogram of a 50-year-old man with a long history of multiple myeloma. The patient presented with acute onset of flank pain and hematuria. The venogram demonstrates a large filling defect within the main renal vein, representing acute renal vein thrombosis. **B** A normal left renal venogram for purposes of comparison. Note that normally there is poor filling of the peripheral branches due to arterial inflow.

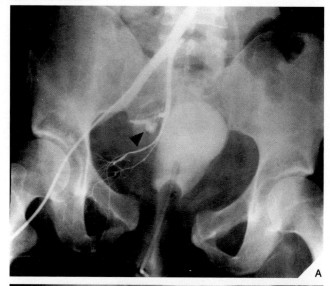

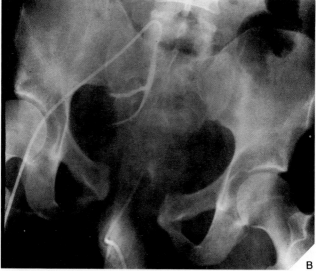

Fig. 3.11 **A** This patient sustained massive injuries in an automobile accident, including a severe diastasis injury to the pelvis. Uncontrolled hemorrhage resulted. An emergency arteriogram demonstrates extravasation from a branch of the right hypogastric artery (*arrow*). **B** Following transcatheter embolization of the traumatized branch, no further extravasation is seen. The patient could then be stabilized clinically. This type of management of massive pelvic hemorrhage has become commonplace.

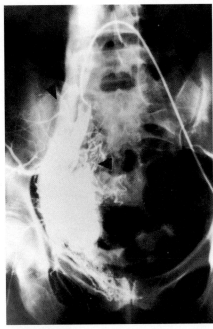

Fig. 3.12 A hypogastric arteriogram demonstrates a large pelvic arteriovenous malformation (*arrow 1*). Note the rapid shunting into the iliac vein (*arrow 2*). This 45-year-old woman presented with lower abdominal pains, and a pulsatile mass on pelvic examination. These lesions are difficult to treat because they are supplied by numerous feeding vessels, and have a marked tendency to progress and recur.

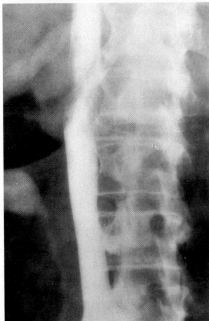

Fig. 3.13 This normal inferior venacavagram demonstrates the characteristic rather featureless appearance of the vessel. The two poorly defined filling defects at the L1 vertebral body level represent the areas of inflow of unopacified blood from each renal vein. The poor definition of these defects as well as the changeability from one film to another allows them to be distinguished from fixed defects, as would be seen with thrombus.

33

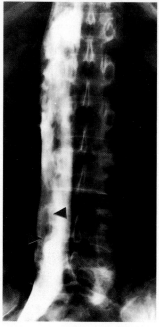

Fig. 3.14 An inferior venacavagram performed from the right iliac vein demonstrates a large radiolucent filling defect occupying the entire length of the vessel. Note the sharply marginated contours (*arrows*), which were constant on all films; this would not be characteristic of a flow-related defect and represents a large thrombus.

4
Selective Abdominal Studies

SELECTIVE VISCERAL ANGIOGRAPHY

The Visceral Circulation (Figs. 4.1–4.3)

The three major aortic branches that supply the gastrointestinal tract in the abdomen are the celiac axis, the superior mesenteric artery, and the inferior mesenteric artery. Normal selective celiac axis, SMA and IMA angiograms are shown in Figs. 4.1–4.3. As in any angiographic study, it is necessary to see the entire sequence of films (arterial, capillary, and venous) to properly evaluate diagnostic findings.

Gastrointestinal Bleeding (Figs. 4.4–4.9)

It has been shown experimentally that angiography can detect bleeding into the GI tract at rates of 0.3 to 1.0 cc per minute or greater.

The most common sites of upper GI bleeding are in the stomach and duodenum, therefore, good opacification of the vessels supplying these regions is imperative, and this includes the left gastric, gastroduodenal, gastroepiploics, splenic, and upper branches of the superior mesenteric artery that supply the duodenum. A site of extravasation is sought which appears as a "puddle," or a dense smudge of contrast persisting after the normal vascular structures are no longer opacified. If the quantity is large enough, this extravasated contrast may outline the mucosal pattern of the gastric or duodenal lumen. Often it is easier to find the bleeding site by first examining late phase films looking for a persistent collection of contrast, if one is found, it can be traced back through earlier phases in order to determine which artery is the source.

Extravasation can be mimicked by dense mucosal staining due to truly hyperemic mucosa, or simply due to a wedged catheter position with over injection of contrast. Generally close inspection of the films will clarify the situation. Another possible pitfall is mistaking the blush of a normal adrenal gland for a site of extravasation. The key to avoiding this error is to note the characteristic shape and location of the adrenal stain. Processes that cause diffuse bleeding, such as hemorrhagic gastritis, usually will not show discrete areas of extravasation, but may demonstrate marked mucosal hyperemia.

Venous bleeding, from esophageal or gastric varices, will not be definitively demonstrated on celiac angiography. The diagnosis can be suggested, however, when the arterial phase does not show a bleeding site, but venous phase films reveal evidence of portal hypertension, such as varices or hepatofugal flow.

Lower GI bleeding (distal to the duodenum) is difficult to monitor clinically because there is no diagnostic procedure for the area equivalent to passing an NG tube. The nature of the bleeding may range from melena to bright red blood per rectum. While the appearance of the blood may provide a clue to the level of the bleeding site, it is also largely dependent on the rate of bleeding. Thus an angiographic study for lower GI bleeding should include not only the inferior and superior mesenteric arteries, but the celiac axis as well, as a bleed from a duodenal source can mimic a lower GI bleed. Profuse lower GI bleeding is associated most often with colonic diverticuli. Other causes include arteriovenous malformations (AVM) or angiodysplasia, ulceration, Meckel's diverticulum, ischemia, and, occasionally, tumors. A diverticular source can be suggested specifically when the extravasated contrast remains in a sharply defined rounded collection on late films, reflecting puddling in the diverticulum itself.

Angiodysplasias are small submucosal vascular malformations that occur in the colon, most often in the cecum. They tend to occur in older patients who may have a history of repeated episodic hemorrhage, or slow continuous GI blood loss. The etiology of angiodysplasias remains a mystery, but there appears to be a significant association with aortic valve disease and conditions in which there is chronic poor cardiac output. Angiographically the lesions usually appear as a small tangle of abnormal arteries with shunting into mesenteric veins; often the easiest way to spot them is to look for these early draining veins first. In a significant percentage of cases these malformations are multiple, so that the entire lower GI tract should be studied if one lesion is found. Due to their small size and submucosal location, angiodysplasias may be almost invisible at surgery, and special preparation of the specimen is necessary to find them pathologically.

Transcatheter therapy has assumed a major role in the management of GI bleeding. One approach consists of infusing a vasoconstrictor, such as vasopressin, directly into the vessels shown to be the source of bleeding (see Fig. 4.8). While this method for the containment of bleeding can be quite effective, it requires maintaining the catheter in place for hours or days, which can result in a considerable management problem. This technique will not be effective if the bleeding vessels are incapable of vasoconstriction, as in some inflammatory and neoplastic conditions. Also, the use of vasoconstricting drugs may be contraindicated in patients with severe coronary artery disease. An alternative technique is transcatheter embolization, in which a device or substance is inserted through the catheter to occlude the bleeding vessel (see Fig. 4.4). This approach has the advantage of producing immediate results, and avoiding the need for an in-dwelling catheter. The extensive collateral circulation of the upper GI tract minimizes the risk of tissue ischemia following embolization.

Embolization and infusion of vasoconstrictors are used in the management of lower GI bleeding as well, but the risk of ischemia after embolization is significantly higher than in the upper GI tract due to the much poorer collateral supply.

Lesions Impairing Visceral Flow (Figs. 4.10–4.13)

Impaired blood flow in the visceral circulation may be acute or chronic. When acute, the results are catastrophic if diagnosis and treatment are not carried out within hours of the onset of symptoms. On the other hand, chronic visceral occlusive disease is tolerated fairly well by most patients, who often present with nonspecific abdominal complaints of many years duration.

The most frequent cause of acute intestinal ischemia is an arterial embolus, usually of cardiac origin. These patients typically present with acute abdominal pain and tenderness, bloody diarrhea, and abdominal distension due to ileus. If there is a history of cardiac arrhythmia, embolus should be strongly suspected and emergency angiography performed. Biplane aortography should be done first, to visualize the origins of the visceral trunks in the lateral view prior to any attempt at selective catheterization, which could cause a proximal embolus to fragment and shower more distally.

Acute ischemia also may be seen in patients with severely compromised cardiac output, "low flow state," or intense vasoconstriction due to other causes. This entity is referred to as "nonocclusive mesenteric ischemia," and may show a characteristic appearance of diffusely narrowed and beaded mesenteric branches. In addition to correcting the low-flow state, infusion of vasodilators directly into a catheter in the superior mesenteric artery may result in marked clinical improvement.

Patients with severe atherosclerosis often have involvement of the proximal visceral trunks. Since the involvement is a gradual process, there is time for collateral circulation to develop. We have encountered asymptomatic patients in whom the celiac and superior mesenteric origins were completely occluded, and the visceral circulation was carried only by a hypertrophied inferior mesenteric artery. Obviously a patient whose entire GI tract is being supplied by only one of these trunks will suffer disastrous intestinal ischemia if that trunk occludes.

"Celiac axis compression syndrome" is a controversial entity that is described most often in young, thin female patients who complain of upper abdominal symptoms (pain, diarrhea) following meals. The symptoms may be so distressing that considerable weight loss occurs. On physical examination, an upper abdominal bruit is audible, and angiography shows a marked extrinsic impression on the superior aspect of the main celiac trunk. This narrowing is due to a crossing diaphragmatic ligament, which can be released surgically without much difficulty. The controversy surrounding this syndrome concerns whether the symptoms are in fact related to the arterial narrowing, although many patients do report relief of symptoms after surgery.

ABDOMINAL TUMORS

Tumors of the abdominal organs vary widely in angiographic appearance. Some lesions are detectable by their abnormal internal vasculature; these abnormal arteries are referred to as "tumor vessels" or "neovascularity." Tumor vessels may have a bizarre appearance, with failure to taper normally, sharp angulations, contrast puddling or staining, and, in some cases, arteriovenous shunting. Some tumors, particularly pancreatic carcinoma, show no significant intrinsic vascularity, but are discovered because of their effect on arteries and veins in the region (encasement). The degree of vascularity does not denote whether the tumor is benign or malignant, but certain patterns are characteristic and will be discussed in the sections on individual abdominal organs.

Liver: Benign and Malignant Tumors (Figs. 4.14–4.21)

Benign lesions that are commonly encountered in the liver include cysts, cavernous hemangiomas, focal nodular hyperplasia, and hepatic adenomas.

Cysts are not true neoplasms, and are rarely of clinical significance; the widespread use of CT and ultrasound has shown them to be much more common than previously thought.

Cavernous hemangiomas are the most common benign neoplasm of the liver. Rarely symptomatic unless they bleed or rupture, generally they do not require specific therapy. The diagnosis can be confirmed almost always by CT, but the angiographic appearance is characteristic.

Focal nodular hyperplasia is a benign hamartomatous lesion composed of normal liver tissue, fibrous septae, and numerous blood vessels. These lesions are generally asymptomatic, most often encountered in young women, and may be single or multiple.

Hepatic adenomas are benign neoplasms, but they may bleed spontaneously, sometimes presenting as a free intra-abdominal hemorrhage. There seems to be an increased incidence of these lesions in women who have taken oral contraceptives. Unlike focal nodular hyperplasia, these lesions are usually solitary, and may be extremely large. Pathologically, they are composed of hepatocytes, but show no bile ducts or Kupffer cells. Unlike focal nodular hyperplasia these lesions never show uptake on radiocolloid liver scans, due to the absence of Kupffer cells.

Metastatic disease is the most frequently encountered malignant process in the liver. The lesions may be single, but are more often multiple, a finding that strongly suggests the diagnosis. While the majority of the blood supply for normal hepatic parenchyma is derived from the portal circulation, metastatic lesions and most primary malignant liver tumors are supplied by the hepatic arterial circulation. Metastatic lesions vary in angiographic appearance; their degree of vascularity is largely determined by the type of primary tumor.

Primary liver tumors (hepatomas) are variable in their angiographic appearance also, but tend to be large and hypervascular, often showing marked hypertrophy of the feeding arteries. A distinctive finding that is highly suggestive of this diagnosis is shunting from the hepatic arteries to the portal veins (arterioportal shunting). This shunting may result in portal hypertension.

Spleen (Fig. 4.22)
The spleen may be affected by trauma, infection, tumor, or infarction. All of these conditions are more appropriately studied by CT or ultrasound than angiography, at least initially. Angiographically the normal spleen appears as a rounded triangular organ, tucked under the diaphragm, in the left upper quadrant. The splenic artery is frequently tortuous, quite commonly showing atherosclerotic calcification in old-

er patients, as well as occasional aneurysm formation.

The venous phase of the splenic arteriogram shows opacification of the splenic vein, which is part of the portal system. The splenic vein is large, and its course is straight, unlike the undulating splenic artery. Since the splenic vein is in intimate contact with the pancreas, it is often affected by abnormalities in this organ, particularly inflammation or neoplasm.

Splenic rupture can be diagnosed by angiography (formerly the "gold standard"), but lobulation and other normal variants in the configuration of the spleen may result in both false positive and negative studies.

The spleen may be involved by primary or metastatic neoplasms as well as diffusely infiltrated in leukemias or lymphomas. The angiographic findings tend to be nonspecific; however, masses, splenic enlargement, or stretching of intrasplenic vessels may be seen.

Pancreas (Figs. 4.23–4.28)

Until fairly recently, angiography was one of the only techniques available for imaging the pancreas. Other imaging modalities have largely replaced angiography, but it remains a useful method of study for delineating regional vascular anatomy, and determining potential resectability of pancreatic carcinoma prior to surgery.

The pancreas receives its blood supply from the celiac axis and superior mesenteric arteries. The head of the gland is supplied by the pancreaticoduodenal arteries, which originate from both the gastroduodenal (a celiac branch) and the superior mesenteric arteries. The body of the pancreas is supplied by the dorsal pancreatic artery, a small vessel which originates usually from the inferior aspect of the celiac axis itself. A series of small arteries arise from the splenic artery inferiorly, which supply the distal body and tail of the pancreas. The largest of these branches is termed the pancreatic magna. All three of these sources contribute to form the transverse pancreatic artery, which runs through the middle of the gland.

Adenocarcinoma, the most common malignant pancreatic tumor, is almost always hypovascular or avascular on angiography. Adenocarcinoma is detected by its effect on normal vessels in the pancreas and the surrounding region. The angiographic term for this effect is "encasement," referring to tubular narrowing, loss of normal tapering, abrupt angulation, and sometimes complete occlusion. The vessels involved depend on the location of the tumor within the pancreas, and may include intrapancreatic, gastroduodenal, splenic, and common hepatic arteries, superior mesenteric branches, and sometimes the main celiac or superior mesenteric trunks themselves. Tumor encasement must be distinguished from atherosclerotic or inflammatory involvement, which can have a similar appearance. Inflammation, particularly pancreatitis, can also produce vascular abnormalities that resemble the changes seen with neoplasm, and differentiation may not always be possible.

The portal venous phase is probably the most important part of the radiologic examination if carcinoma of the pancreas is suspected. The splenic and proximal superior mesenteric veins have an intimate anatomical relationship to the pancreas. These venous structures are more compressible than the arteries, usually resulting in an angiographically detectable effect of a tumor on the veins before any arterial abnormalities are apparent. Venous involvement ranges from encasement to complete occlusion, which is commonly seen in advanced lesions.

Other tumors that occur in the pancreas include islet cell tumors, which may or may not be endocrinologically active, cystadenomas, cystadenocarcinomas, and metastatic disease.

Stomach, Small And Large Intestine (Fig. 4.29)

There are more effective and less invasive means of diagnosing most neoplasms of the GI tract than angiography, so it is seldom used for this purpose. One situation in which it may be useful, though, is in an investigation of occult GI bleeding. Ulceration of submucosal tumors in the stomach or small bowel may be extremely difficult to detect on barium studies, CT, or endoscopy. Leiomyomas in particular are often quite vascular, and may be associated with massive intermittent GI bleeding.

Angiodysplasias of the colon are malformations rather than neoplasms and are discussed under Selective Visceral Angiography.

Kidneys (Figs. 4.30–4.35)

The most common mass encountered in the kidney is the simple cyst, a benign lesion usually discovered incidentally. Ultrasound is the best study to confirm the diagnosis, but angiographic findings are also distinctive.

Benign solid neoplasms of the kidney, which include adenomas, onocytomas, and angiomyolipomas, are relatively rare, and may be difficult or impossible to distinguish angiographically from renal cancer, although certain features may be suggestive.

Hypernephroma, or renal cell carcinoma, is the most frequent malignant tumor of the kidney. Most of these tumors have a characteristic angiographic appearance consisting of enlarged feeding arteries, marked hypervascularity, arteriovenous shunting, and, in some cases, extension of tumor into the renal vein and inferior vena cava. These lesions may be very large, with flow so rapid that two or three times the normal contrast injection rate and volume is required for adequate opacification. Since renal vein involvement is common, the venous phase must be evaluated carefully, and if there is any question direct study of the inferior vena cava and renal vein should be performed. Some hypernephromas are hypovascular or almost entirely avascular, and may be associated with a cystic component.

Transitional cell carcinoma is generally hypovascular on angiography; however the arteries in the region of the tumor may show evidence of spreading, infiltration, or encasements.

Adrenals (Figs. 4.36, 4.37)

With a few exceptions, computed tomography and ultrasound have replaced angiography as the imaging modality of choice in the diagnosis of adrenal disease. The adrenal glands receive their blood supply from three sources: the renal artery, the aorta, and the inferior phrenic artery. The small caliber of these vessels coupled with the fact that all must be injected to completely outline the anatomy of the gland result in an examination that is prolonged and tedious.

In the past, adrenal venography has been used extensively to investigate adrenal abnormalities. The technique, which is quite difficult, offers the advantage of obtaining adrenal vein samples that are diagnostic in many hormone secreting adrenal tumors. A distinct risk of adrenal venography is rupture of the capsule of the gland, which results in irreversible ablation of function. This has also been done intentionally in some conditions to produce a nonsurgical adrenalectomy.

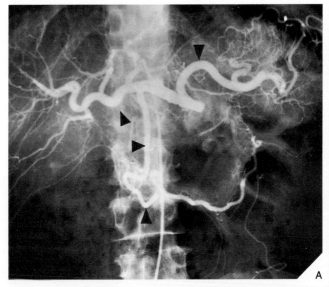

Fig. 4.1 **A** An arterial-phase film from a selective celiac axis injection. The examination demonstrates the splenic (*arrow* 1), hepatic (*arrow* 2), gastroduodenal (*arrow* 3), and the gastroepiploic (*arrow* 4) arteries as well as branches of these vessels. Small omental vessels are demonstrated also (*arrow* 5). **B** A mucosal-phase film from the same injection demonstrates diffuse

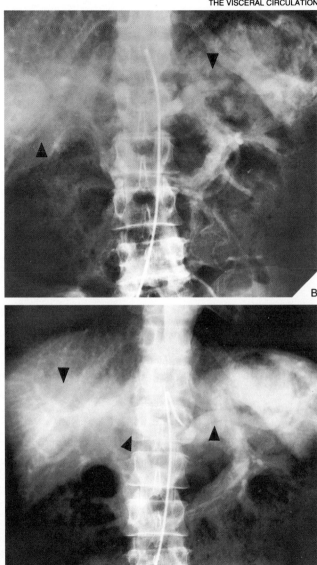

B

C

opacification of the liver (*arrow* 1) and spleen parenchyma (*arrow* 2) as well as a mucosal blush over the stomach. **C** The late phase, or portal phase, of the same injection, demonstrates opacification of the splenic vein (*arrow* 1), portal vein (*arrow* 2), and intrahepatic portal circulation (*arrow* 3).

45

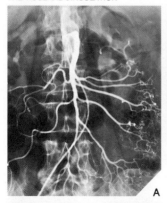

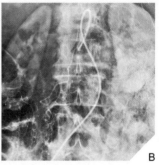

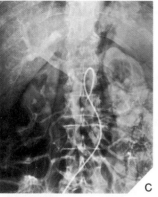

Fig. 4.2 **A** An arterial-phase film from a selective study of the superior mesenteric artery demonstrates this vessel originating anteriorly from the abdominal aorta at the level of the T12–L1 disc space. The vessel supplies the duodenum, jejunum, ileum, and the proximal colon. **B** A capillary-phase film from the superior mesenteric artery injection demonstrates the normal diffuse mucosal blush of the small intestine. **C** The venous-phase film demonstrates opacification of the branch mesenteric, the superior mesenteric, and the main portal veins.

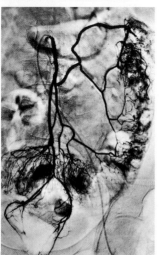

Fig. 4.3 A selective study of the inferior mesenteric artery, which generally originates anteriorly and slightly directed to the left at the L3–4 disc space level. This is a subtraction film, which shows the arterial branching more clearly. Note that the circulation to the left colon is considerably more sparse than in the superior mesenteric distribution. The rectum is supplied by both the inferior mesenteric artery branches of the hypogastric arteries.

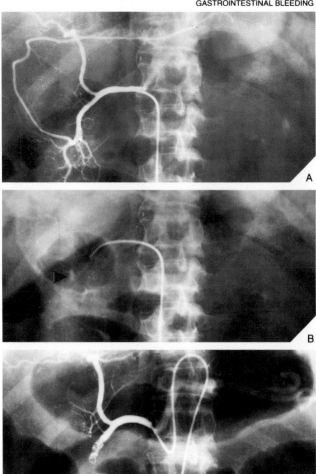

Fig. 4.4 **A** A 76-year-old man presented with massive upper GI bleeding suspected to be of duodenal origin. An early film of a selective injection into the gastroduodenal artery demonstrates the normal appearance of the duodenal branches. **B** The later-phase film of the same injection shows a small smudge of contrast (*arrow*) in the region of the duodenum, which represents the site of bleeding. **C** Transcatheter therapy was used to manage this hemorrhage. Several stainless steel coils were inserted through the catheter to occlude the gastroduodenal artery. This follow-up arteriogram shows no further filling of the midportion of the gastroduodenal artery, and no further extravasation. The bleeding stopped promptly. Generally this type of embolization in the upper GI tract is quite safe due to the rich collateral blood supply of the upper abdominal organs.

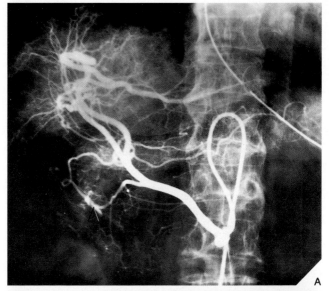

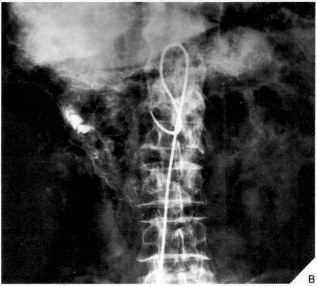

Fig. 4.5 A patient presented with massive upper GI bleeding of duodenal origin. **A** The arterial-phase film demonstrates an irregular collection of contrast beginning to appear next to one of the duodenal branches (*arrow*). **B** The later-phase film demonstrates a large puddle of extravasation outlining the mucosal pattern of the duodenum (*arrow*).

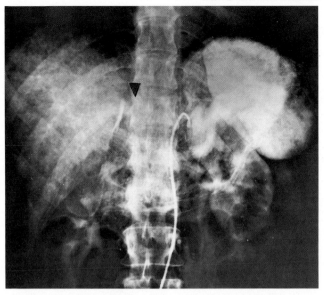

Fig. 4.6 A mucosal-phase film from a celiac study of a patient admitted for upper GI bleeding demonstrates an elongated triangular stain to the right of the T12 vertebral body (*arrow*). The shape and location of this stain is characteristic for the normal blush of the adrenal gland, and should not be confused with a site of extravasation.

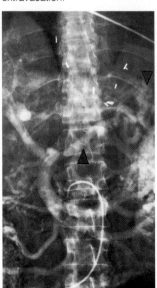

Fig. 4.7 A 47-year-old alcoholic patient presented with massive upper GI bleeding. The celiac and superior mesenteric study showed no evidence of active arterial extravasation, but the venous-phase films demonstrated evidence of severe portal hypertension. This is a venous-phase film from the superior mesenteric injection, demonstrating hepatofugal flow into the splenic vein as well as filling of gastric varices (*arrows*). In this type of situation the findings are strongly suggestive of a venous source of bleeding.

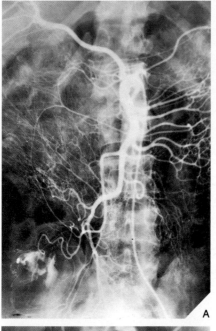

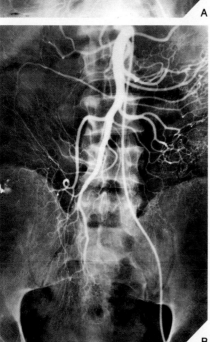

Fig. 4.8 **A** This is a superior mesenteric arteriogram of a 59-year-old patient with massive lower GI bleeding. The examination demonstrates gross extravasation of contrast in the cecum. The primary point of extravasation is a sharply-defined rounded collection of contrast, which represents a diverticulum. In this case, an attempt was made to control the bleeding by infusing vasopressin directly into the catheter in the superior mesenteric artery. **B** A follow-up film demonstrates diffuse vasoconstriction and a considerably reduced amount of extravasation in the cecum, although some puddling remains.

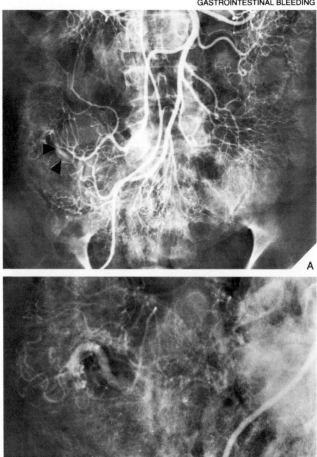

Fig. 4.9 **A** Superior mesenteric arteriogram of a 66-year-old man with chronic congestive failure and recurrent episodes of massive lower GI bleeding demonstrates a subtle abnormality in the region of the cecum. If this region is examined closely, an early draining vein can be seen (*arrows*). **B** A magnified view of this area in a slightly later phase shows more clearly this early draining vein. The findings are characteristic for an angiodysplasia of the colon, a specific type of vascular malformation. These are most often found in the cecum, although they may be located anywhere in the colon, and may be multiple.

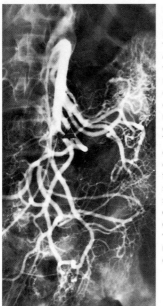

Fig. 4.10 A 76-year-old man presented with acute abdominal pain and diarrhea following aortic valve replacement and cardioversion for arterial fibrillation. The superior mesenteric arteriogram demonstrates a large filling defect within the superior mesenteric artery (*arrow*), extending into several branches. The findings are quite characteristic for an acute embolus. When embolization to the visceral circulation is suspected, the initial study should be a biplane aortogram in order to rule out the presence of emboli at the origins of the vessels, which could shower more distally on attempted catheterization.

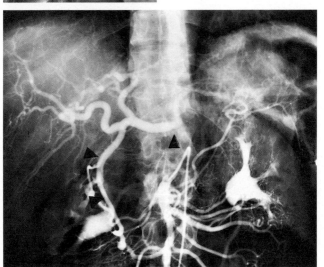

Fig. 4.11 A superior mesenteric artery injection demonstrates filling of the celiac axis through the gastroduodenal collateral pathway (*arrows*). This type of filling is seen when there is a high grade stenosis or complete occlusion of the proximal celiac trunk. Due to good collateral reconstitution, this type of occlusive process is often asymptomatic.

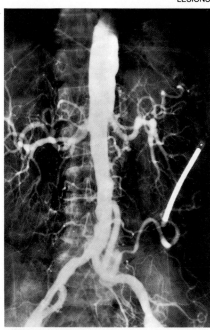

Fig. 4.12 Aortogram of a 58-year-old woman with diffuse atherosclerosis and complaints of abdominal pain after eating. The film demonstrates poor filling of the celiac axis, no filling of the superior mesenteric artery, and filling of a hypertrophied inferior mesenteric trunk (*arrow*). The entire visceral circulation can be carried by any one of these three visceral trunks if the process develops slowly, and adequate collateral pathways develop.

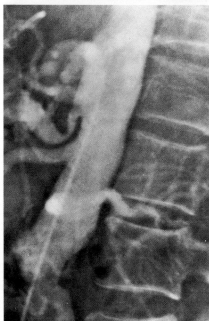

Fig. 4.13 A lateral view of a flush aortogram demonstrates the origins of the celiac and superior mesenteric arteries. The proximal celiac trunk shows a sharp impression on its superior margin, with poststenotic dilation. This finding is characteristic for celiac axis compression due to a crossing diaphragmatic ligament. The relationship of this finding to upper abdominal symptomatology is controversial.

53

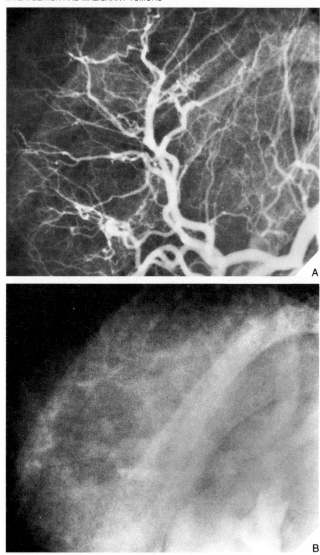

Fig. 4.14 A defect in the right lobe of the liver can be seen on a liver spleen scan in a 35-year-old woman with a history of lymphoma. (This case occurred before the era of computed tomography.) **A** The arterial phase demonstrates minimal stretching of the intrahepatic arteries, with no evidence of abnormal vascularity. **B** The hepatogram, or parenchymal phase of the study shows a sharply marginated round avascular area. These findings are compatible with a simple cyst of the liver.

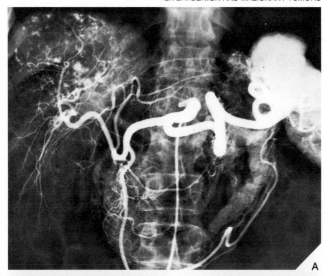

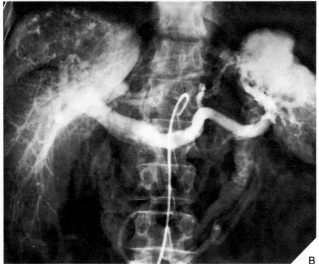

Fig. 4.15 A 70-year-old woman was found to have a large mass in the right lobe of the liver on sonography and computed tomography. **A** The celiac axis injection demonstrates numerous small puddles of contrast on the periphery of the lesion. **B** The late phase of the examination shows opacification of the portal system with persistent dense puddling of contrast in the right lobe lesion. Such puddling with prolonged stasis is quite characteristic for benign cavernous hemangioma. This type of lesion is generally asymptomatic and requires no specific therapy.

55

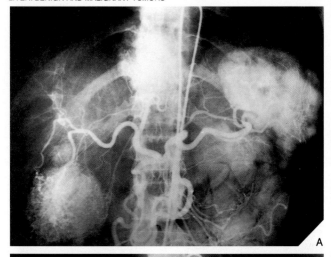

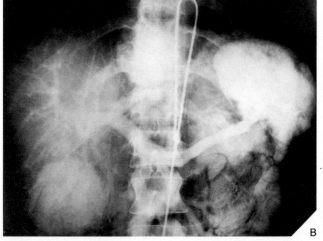

Fig. 4.16 Computed tomography and ultrasonography demonstrated a mass in the right lobe of the liver in this 38-year-old woman who was admitted complaining of dull right upper quadrant pain. **A** The arteriogram demonstrates a large round hypervascular mass extending from the inferior aspect of the right lobe. There is an enlarged feeding artery with a faint radiating pattern of internal vasculature seen. No arteriovenous shunting is present. Also note the presence of a common origin of the celiac and superior mesenteric arteries, a normal variant. **B** The late phase of the same injection demonstrates good opacification of the portal system and dense staining of the rounded liver lesion. These findings are quite consistent with focal nodular hyperplasia, a benign harmartomatous lesion.

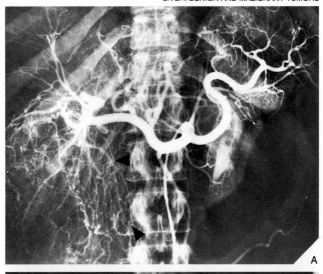

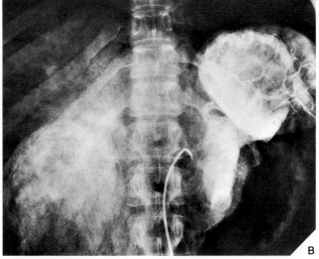

Fig. 4.17 **A** Hepatic adenomas, like focal nodular hyperplasia, are usually encountered in young women. Hepatic adenomas may bleed spontaneously, as occurred in this 28-year-old woman who presented with free intra-abdominal hemorrhage. The celiac axis injection demonstrates a large hypervascular mass involving the inferior aspect of the right lobe of the liver. Numerous bizarre blood vessels are noted within the mass, with no discernible organized pattern. **B** A late-phase film demonstrates the large hypervascular mass, with a defect at its inferior margin most likely representing the area of hemorrhage. These lesions have been associated with oral contraceptive intake.

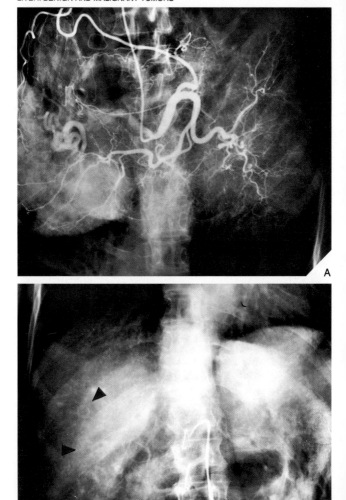

Fig. 4.18 A 62-year-old woman with a history of colon resection for carcinoma presented with a rising CEA titer. Computed tomography showed some inhomogeneity, but no definite lesions. **A** The celiac arteriogram does not demonstrate significant arterial abnormalities in the liver. **B** The hepatogram phase, however, demonstrates several round avascular lesions with moderately vascular rims. This hypovascular type of lesion is commonly associated with colon, breast, and lung carcinoma primaries.

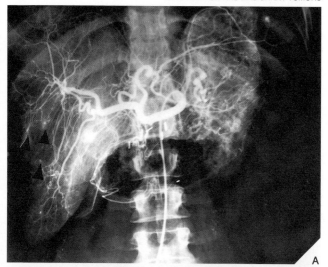

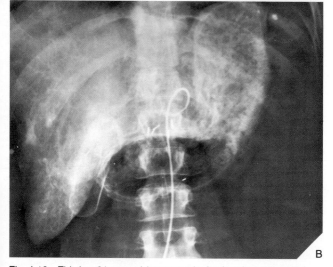

Fig. 4.19 This is a 31-year-old woman who had undergone a total pancreatectomy for a functioning islet cell tumor one year previously. She now presented with a recurrence of symptoms. **A** The celiac injection demonstrates multiple hypervascular lesions scattered throughout the right lobe of the liver. **B** The late-phase film shows these lesions more clearly. Hypervascular metastatic lesions tend to be associated with hypernephromas, some sarcomas, carcinoid, primary endocrine, and, occasionally, colon tumors. The thin-walled curvilinear structure overlapping the inferior edge of the right lobe of the liver represents the blush of the normal gallbladder wall.

59

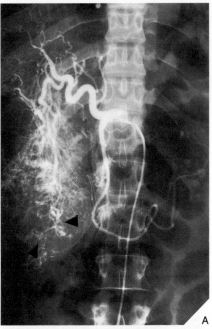

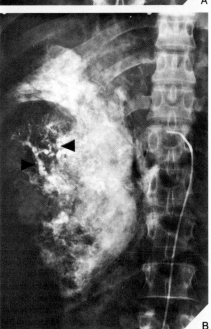

Fig. 4.20 A 39-year-old male with a ten-year history of chronic active hepatitis presented with a large abdominal mass. **A** Celiac arteriography demonstrated the mass to be of hepatic origin. The bizarre tumor vessels (*arrows*) are quite characteristic for a malignant tumor such as hepatoma. **B** The late-phase film demonstrates filling of intrahepatic portal vein radicles (*arrows*). Portal venous radicles would not fill from a hepatic arterial injection, normally, and this type of arterial-portal shunting is quite characteristic of hepatoma.

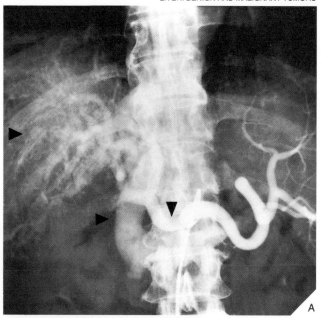

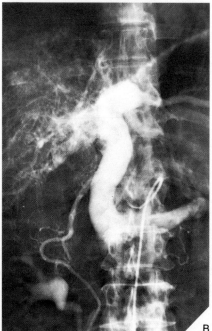

Fig. 4.21 This 72-year-old Chinese man presented with massive upper GI bleeding. **A** The celiac arteriogram demonstrates a large hypervascular mass occupying most of the liver (*arrow* 1). There is massive shunting from the hepatic artery (*arrow* 2) directly into the main portal vein (*arrow* 3). **B** The later-phase film demonstrates further filling of the portal vein and hepatofugal flow, which is responsible for the variceal bleeding. This type of shunting into the portal system with variceal bleeding may be encountered in large hepatomas.

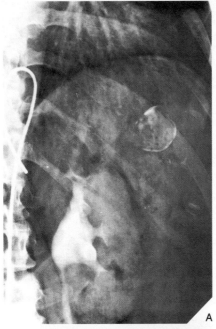

Fig. 4.22 A When a 45-year-old woman had abdominal films taken to evaluate back pain, a rounded curvilinear calcification was noted incidentally in the left upper quadrant. This type of calcification is quite typical of that seen in blood vessels, particularly aneurysms. B A splenic arteriogram demonstrates a large aneurysm in the hilus of the spleen, which corresponds to the area of calcification (*arrows*). The splenic artery is affected by atherosclerosis, frequently, and often shows areas of calcification within its walls.

A

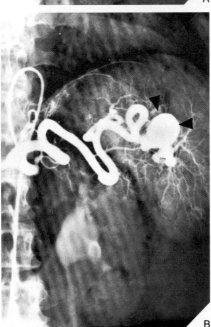

B

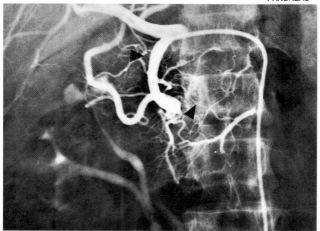

Fig. 4.23 An injection into the gastroduodenal artery (*arrow* 1) demonstrates the normal pancreaticoduodenal arteries that supply the head of the pancreas (*arrow* 2). The superior mesenteric artery also contributes to this circulation.

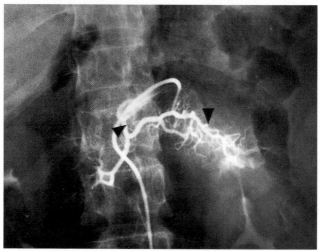

Fig. 4.24 The catheter tip is in the pancreatic magna, a branch of the splenic artery. Injection fills the transverse pancreatic artery (*arrow* 1), and there is retrograde filling of the dorsal pancreatic artery, (*arrow* 2), a branch of the main celiac trunk. No abnormalities are seen on this particular study. Angiographically, the pancreas is not a very vascular organ. Often the capillary phase of a good quality celiac arteriogram will show a faint parenchymal blush of the organ, particularly in the body and tail. The pancreatic head is frequently difficult to distinguish from the mucosal blush of the intimately associated duodenal sweep.

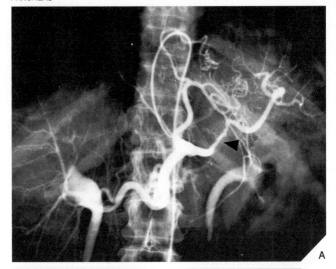

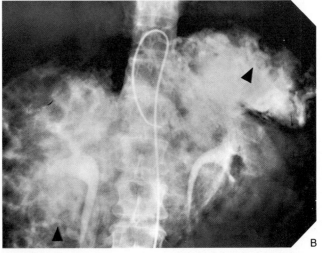

Fig. 4.25 A Celiac axis study of a 61-year-old man, who presented with abdominal pain and weight loss. The film demonstrates irregular narrowing of the midportion of the splenic artery (*arrow*). This type of tubular narrowing is referred to as "encasement," and is characteristic of involvement of blood vessels by a malignant process. **B** The late-phase film does not demonstrate opacification of the splenic vein, which has been completely occluded by the tumor. Collateral vessels may be noted in the region of the spleen (*arrow* 1). Also visible are numerous hypovascular masses within the liver (*arrow* 2), representing widespread metastatic liver disease. The findings are classic for pancreatic adenocarcinoma with liver metastasis.

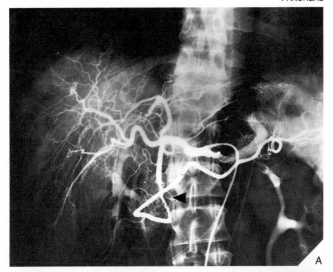

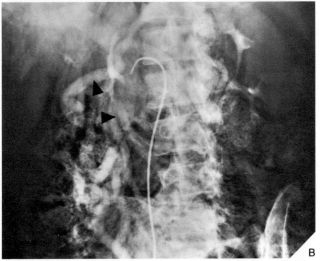

Fig. 4.26 This 49-year-old man presented with abdominal pain and weight loss. Computed tomography showed a mass in the uncinate process of the pancreas. Angiography was performed to evaluate the potential for resectability. **A** The common hepatic artery injection demonstrates a long narrowed segment of the distal gastroduodenal artery (*arrows*), but no other significant abnormalities. **B** The venous phase of the superior mesenteric artery injection demonstrates occlusion of the superior mesenteric vein (*arrow* 1), with filling of collateral venous channels (*arrow* 2). This type of major venous encasement implies the presence of an unresectable tumor.

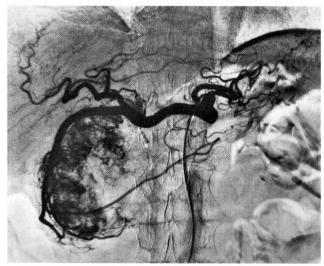

Fig. 4.27 Islet cell tumors of the pancreas may or may not be endocrinologically active. Tumors that actively secrete hormone tend to be diagnosed when quite small due to the severe clinical symptomatology. Nonfunctioning islet cell tumors often reach a large size before being detected. In this case, the patient presented with a palpable abdominal mass. The arteriogram demonstrates a huge hypervascular mass in the head of the pancreas. The gastroduodenal artery is enlarged, and it is draped around the mass. Islet cell tumors, whether functioning or nonfunctioning, tend to be hypervascular.

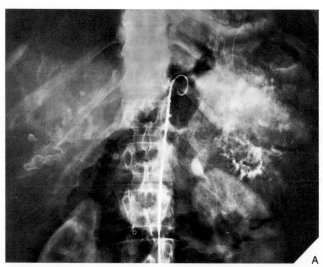

A

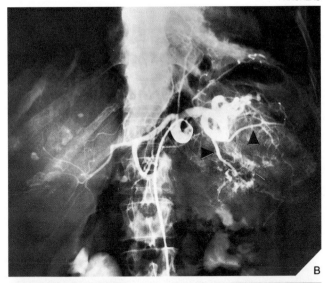

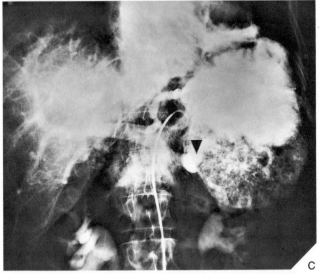

Fig. 4.28 Cystadenomas and cystadenocarcinomas frequently reach a large size before clinical detection also. As their names imply both contain cystic and solid elements, and both frequently show internal calcification, often in a stellate pattern. Although the diagnosis of "cystadenoma–cystadenocarcinoma" is not difficult to make due to its distinctive appearance on CT, ultrasound, and angiography (A, B, C), it is generally impossible to determine whether a lesion is malignant or not prior to surgery.

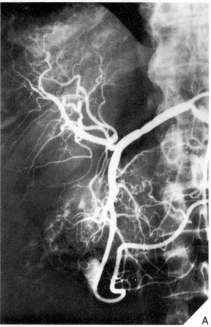

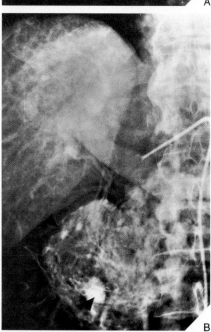

Fig. 4.29 This patient presented with intermittent upper GI bleeding and negative endoscopy. **A** This common hepatic injection demonstrates a large hypervascular mass supplied by gastroduodenal branches. **B** The late-phase film shows fairly dense staining. (*arrows*). At surgery, this lesion was found to be a gastric leiomyoma. These lesions may involve the stomach or the small intestine, and can be the cause of intermittent massive GI bleeding.

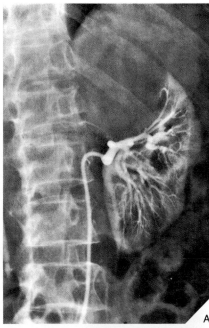

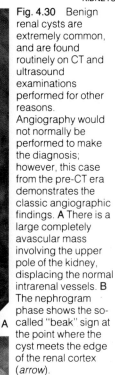

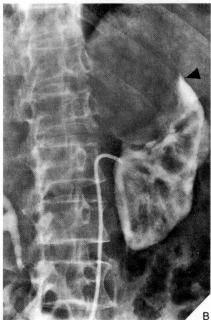

Fig. 4.30 Benign renal cysts are extremely common, and are found routinely on CT and ultrasound examinations performed for other reasons. Angiography would not normally be performed to make the diagnosis; however, this case from the pre-CT era demonstrates the classic angiographic findings. **A** There is a large completely avascular mass involving the upper pole of the kidney, displacing the normal intrarenal vessels. **B** The nephrogram phase shows the so-called "beak" sign at the point where the cyst meets the edge of the renal cortex (*arrow*).

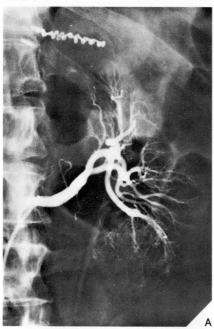

Fig. 4.31 A, B
Oncocytomas are benign renal parenchymal lesions that are often indistinguishable from hypernephromas prior to surgery. Features that suggest this diagnosis include a sharply marginated round shape, a relatively uniform consistency, and, in many cases, the stellate pattern of vessels within the lesion. This case demonstrates a typical oncocytoma involving the lower pole of the left kidney. A heminephrectomy was performed.

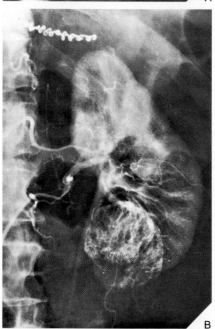

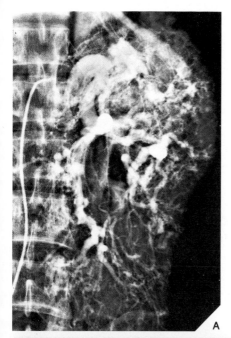

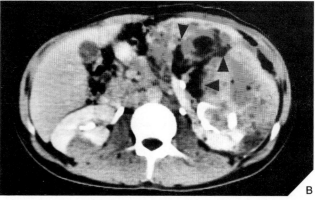

Fig. 4.32 A 24-year-old man, known to have tuberous sclerosis presented with acute abdominal pain on the left side, and a dropping hematocrit. **A** The arteriogram demonstrates a huge hypervascular mass involving almost the entire left kidney, with enlarged feeding vessels and pseudoaneurysms, but no evidence of arteriovenous shunting. **B** The CT scan shows clearly the large amount of fat within the lesion (*arrows*), a finding that is pathognomonic for angiomyolipoma, a common lesion in patients with tuberous sclerosis. Though these lesions are benign, they may bleed massively, necessitating nephrectomy.

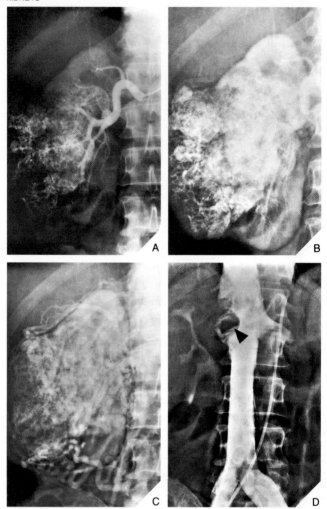

Fig. 4.33 Hypernephroma, or renal cell carcinoma, is the most common malignant tumor of the kidney. In most cases, this lesion has a highly characteristic appearance as is illustrated in this 58-year-old man who presented with painless gross hematuria. **A, B** The arteriograms demonstrate a very large, profusely hypervascular mass occupying the midportion of the kidney. **C** The late-phase film demonstrates filling of numerous collateral veins, suggesting renal vein obstruction on the basis of tumor invasion. **D** This is confirmed by direct inferior venacavography, which shows the tumor thrombus protruding from the right renal vein orifice into the lumen of the cava (*arrow*). Extension of a tumor into the renal vein is seen commonly, and the tumor thrombus may extend as high as the right atrium.

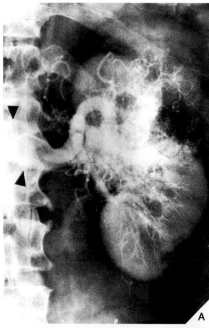

Fig. 4.34 This patient presented with a large hypernephroma involving the left kidney. In this case, there is rapid arteriovenous shunting through the tumor, rather than renal vein invasion. **A** On the arterial injection almost immediate opacification of the renal vein (*arrows*) can be appreciated. **B** A later-phase film demonstrates the presence of periureteral collateral veins (*arrows*), due to the increased venous pressure caused by the arteriovenous shunting.

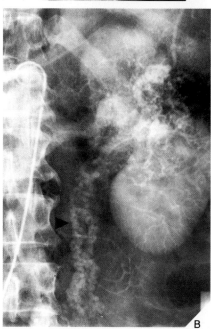

73

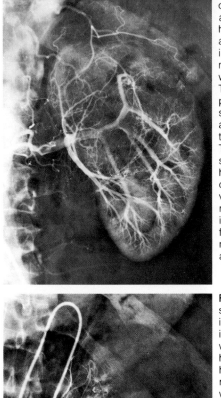

Fig. 4.35 Unlike renal cell carcinoma, transitional cell carcinoma generally appears hypovascular on angiography, as seen in this 72-year-old man who presented with gross hematuria. The retrograde pyelogram (not shown) demonstrated a large mass filling the left renal pelvis. The arteriogram shows a hypovascular mass displacing the blood vessels around the renal pelvis. If the film is examined closely, a fine pattern of neovascularity can be appreciated.

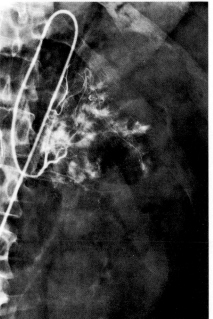

Fig. 4.36 A selective study of the left inferior adrenal artery in a 46-year-old man with a three-year history of hypertension, and a recent 40 pound weight loss. The study demonstrates a large hypovascular mass involving the adrenal gland. At surgery this was found to be an adrenal cortical carcinoma.

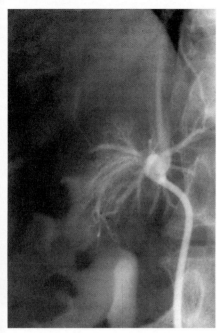

Fig. 4.37 A normal adrenal venogram. Adrenal venography can be used to evaluate changes in the architecture of a gland as well as to obtain venous samples for evaluating hormone secretion. Adrenal vein sampling is difficult to perform and is somewhat hazardous as overdistension of the veins can result in capsular rupture and loss of glandular function.

5
The Extremities

ARTERIOGRAPHY

Modern vascular surgery would not be possible without high-quality angiography, particularly in the extremities. The most common indication is to evaluate atherosclerosis involving the lower extremities, which may present clinically as claudication (cramping on exercise), pain at rest, or actual gangrene. Arteriography is frequently the key to therapeutic decision making and surgical planning. The angiographer should therefore have at least a basic knowledge of vascular surgery to determine precisely what information is required for each particular case. In planning a surgical approach, it is necessary to see not only the actual sites of pathology (stenosis, occlusion, aneurysm, embolus), but the circulation above and below as well (the inflow and outflow).

Peripheral arteriography is also widely used in the management of suspected vascular trauma. Trauma may result in disruption of vessels with hemorrhage, pseudoaneurysm formation, thrombosis, or extrinsic compression. Early diagnosis and prompt intervention are essential.

Peripheral arteriography is a relatively simple procedure to perform and carries a low complication rate in experienced hands. The contrast medium injected does result in significant discomfort for the patient, and premedication for pain is given routinely. Digital image processing is a recent development that allows arteriography to be performed with either an intravenous contrast injection or a direct arterial injection of much less concentrated contrast material—in either case there is considerably less discomfort. It appears likely that in the near future essentially all arteriography will be performed with some type of digital imaging.

Atherosclerotic Disease (Figs. 5.1–5.4)

Occlusive atherosclerotic disease of the lower extremities is an extremely common clinical problem. Occlusive disease has a definite predilection for certain sites, one of the earliest of which is the superficial femoral artery at the level of the adductor canal. The pattern of the disease shown in Fig. 5.1 is quite common and may be associated with either severe claudication or frank ischemia. The importance of the deep femoral circulation in preserving limb viability is readily apparent. Femoral-popliteal bypass grafting or percutaneous transluminal angioplasty are the usual treatments for this disorder.

Aneurysmal Disease (Figs. 5.5–5.9)

In some patients, atherosclerosis is manifested not by narrowing and occlusion of vessels but by abnormal widening of vessels with eventual progression to frank aneurysm formation. Certain sites are prone to this type of disease, including the lower abdominal aorta and the common femoral and popliteal arteries. Often aneurysms in several of these locations coexist in the same patient. Many aneurysms are picked up incidentally on routine physical examination as pulsatile masses. In other patients, the lesions are first manifested by a complication such as embolization, thrombosis, or rupture.

Arterial Embolism (Figs. 5.10, 5.11)

Emboli in the peripheral circulation are a common cause of acute ischemia. These emboli may originate from the heart, as in atrial fibrillation associated with mural thrombus; they may also originate from a segment of the peripheral circulation and lodge more distally, as in the case of embolization from a popliteal aneurysm shown in Fig. 5.4B. Since these emboli lodge in previously patent vessels, there often is a lack of established collateral blood flow and ischemia may be severe. In addition to demonstrating the site of embolization, it is obviously essential to investigate the source as well.

Arterial Trauma (Figs. 5.12–5.14)

Peripheral arteriography is widely used in the management of suspected vascular trauma and has been partly responsible for the steady improvement in limb salvage rates over the past 20 years. Trauma may result in disruption of blood vessels with hemorrhage or pseudoaneurysm formation, intimal tears, thrombosis, or extrinsic compression. Early diagnosis and prompt intervention are essential. Transcatheter embolization techniques have added a new dimension to the management of some of these patients. In many cases, acute hemorrhage can be controlled by injecting embolic materials through the angiographic catheter, obviating the need for surgery.

Tumors (Fig. 5.15)

Prior to the era of computed tomography, angiography was commonly performed as a preoperative measure in patients with tumors of the extremities. It is now less commonly used, although the information provided can be extremely helpful in planning resection of the lesion while preserving the maximum amount of normal tissue. Because their angiographic appearance is so variable, it is usually impossible to make a precise diagnosis of tumors in the extremities on this basis. The vascularity may range from being almost entirely absent to profuse. In some instances, the tumor causes encasement of the normal arteries and veins in the region. Embolization through the angiographic catheter has been used in some cases either as a palliative measure or to make extremely vascular lesions more resectable.

Arteriovenous Malformation (Figs. 5.16, 5.17)

Abnormal arteriovenous communications may be congenital or secondary to trauma. The communication may be a simple fistula, allowing shunting from an artery into a vein, or it may consist of an extensive tangle of abnormal arteries and veins, resulting in marked disability and deformity. While these lesions are benign by definition, they may be so extensive and progressive that numerous surgical procedures, including amputation, become necessary.

Vasculitis (Fig. 5.18)

The arteriographic findings in vasculitis vary widely and depend on the anatomic sites involved as well as the precise nature of the pathologic process. The distal vessels are most often involved, particularly in the hands and feet. The findings may include distal occlusions and irregular stenoses or "beading." It is important to differentiate fixed narrowing due to vasculitis from transient vascular spasm, which is seen often in arteriography of the hand. The use of intraarterial vasodilators may be necessary to resolve the question.

VENOGRAPHY

Despite the availability of numerous noninvasive imaging techniques, contrast venography remains the "gold standard" in the diagnosis of deep venous thrombosis (DVT). The angiographer quickly develops an appreciation of the difficulties involved in making this diagnosis clinically; certainly every swollen or painful leg does not turn out to be venous thrombosis, and the standard tests for DVT in the physical examination are notoriously unreliable. Since the diagnosis of deep venous thrombosis carries serious clinical implications (i.e., risk of pulmonary embolus) and involves a relatively high-risk type of treatment (anticoagulation), it is essential that the most definitive study possible be obtained.

Lower Extremity Venography (Figs. 5.19–5.26)

Leg venography is a simple study to perform, consisting of an injection of contrast material through an intravenous line in the foot. The risks are the same as those of any study involving contrast media, with a somewhat increased danger of extravasation during the injection. Care must be taken to ensure that the intravenous line is in a good position prior to injection. With newer techniques of performing the study and the use of less concentrated contrast media, patient discomfort is minimal and the previously described complication of "post-venogram phlebitis" is uncommon. The diagnosis of deep venous thrombosis is seldom difficult to make with a good-quality study.

Upper Extremity Venography (Fig. 5.27)

The most common indication for venography in the upper extremity is to evaluate suspected subclavian vein occlusion. This condition can occur spontaneously after extreme muscular exertion, as a complication of central venous catheters, or as a result of extrinsic compression (e.g., by tumor). Upper extremity edema is the most common presenting symptom, and venous engorgement may also be noted.

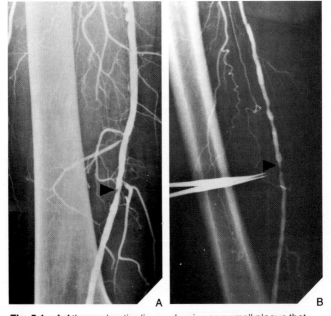

Fig. 5.1 **A** Atherosclerotic disease begins as a small plaque that progressively impinges on the lumen of the vessel (*arrow*), in this case, the superficial femoral artery. At this stage of the disease it is unlikely that significant symptomatology will occur. **B** This view demonstrates progression of the atherosclerotic disease to a tight stenosis (*arrow*). This type of lesion is most often associated with mild claudication on exercise.

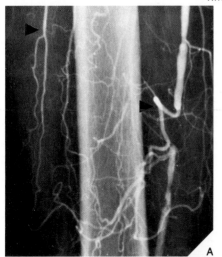

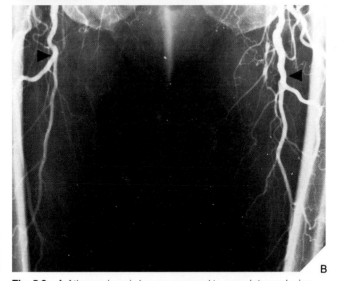

Fig. 5.2 **A** Atherosclerosis has progressed to complete occlusion of one segment of the vessel. Note that the vessel is reconstituted by numerous enlarged collateral vessels from the deep femoral circulation (*arrow* 1) as well as from the termination of the superficial femoral artery (*arrow* 2). This type of finding is also associated with symptoms of exertional pain rather than symptoms at rest. **B** This film of the thighs from a bilateral peripheral arteriogram demonstrates that both superficial femoral arteries are completely occluded. The deep femoral arteries (*arrows*) are hypertrophied and send collaterals down to the distal thighs (*continued on next page*).

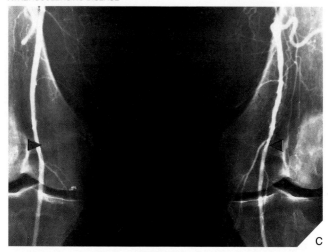

Fig. 5.2 C In the same patient, both distal superficial femoral arteries are reconstituted and fill fairly normal-appearing popliteal arteries (*arrows*).

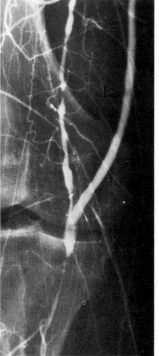

Fig. 5.3 This is an arteriogram of the knee region in a patient who underwent a femoral popliteal bypass graft using a segment of autogenous vein (*arrow*). While the graft still remains open, progression of atherosclerotic disease both above and below the level of graft insertion is likely to cause graft failure due to inadequate flow. Atherosclerosis is a generalized disorder; bypassing one segment of the disease does not stop its progression.

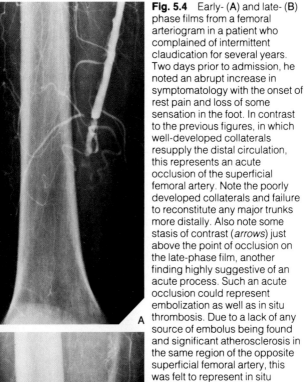

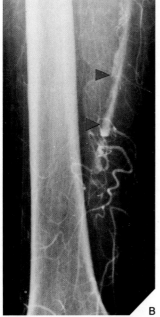

Fig. 5.4 Early- (**A**) and late- (**B**) phase films from a femoral arteriogram in a patient who complained of intermittent claudication for several years. Two days prior to admission, he noted an abrupt increase in symptomatology with the onset of rest pain and loss of some sensation in the foot. In contrast to the previous figures, in which well-developed collaterals resupply the distal circulation, this represents an acute occlusion of the superficial femoral artery. Note the poorly developed collaterals and failure to reconstitute any major trunks more distally. Also note some stasis of contrast (*arrows*) just above the point of occlusion on the late-phase film, another finding highly suggestive of an acute process. Such an acute occlusion could represent embolization as well as in situ thrombosis. Due to a lack of any source of embolus being found and significant atherosclerosis in the same region of the opposite superficial femoral artery, this was felt to represent in situ thrombosis of preexisting disease.

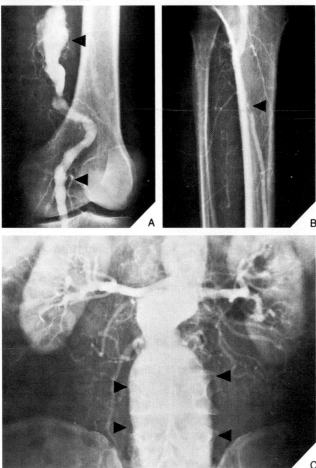

Fig. 5.5 A This 71-year-old man was admitted with acute ischemia of the left foot. On physical examination he was found to have a pulsatile mass just above the knee as well as a pulsatile abdominal mass. This film from a femoral arteriogram demonstrates a very irregular fusiform aneurysm of the distal superficial femoral artery (*arrow* 1) as well as diffuse widening (ectasia) of the popliteal artery (*arrow* 2). **B** The next lower angiographic field demonstrates complete occlusion of the anterior tibial and peroneal arteries and a radiolucent filling defect within the proximal posterior tibial artery (*arrow*), which is pathognomonic of embolization and presumed to originate from the proximal aneurysm. **C** Popliteal aneurysms are frequently bilateral and, in a very high percentage of cases, are associated with abdominal aortic aneurysms, as was the case with this patient (*arrows*). The abdominal aorta should be evaluated in any patient found to have a popliteal aneurysm.

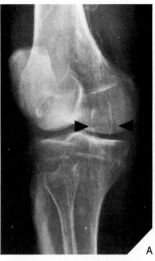 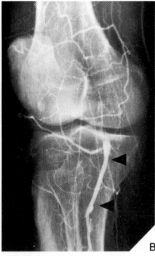

Fig. 5.6 **A** This radiograph demonstrates shell-like calcification of the popliteal artery (*arrows*) in a patient admitted with acute ischemia of the right lower leg. The widened caliber of this calcification compared to a normal popliteal artery suggests the presence of a popliteal aneurysm. **B** The arteriogram demonstrates occlusion of the popliteal artery at the knee with collateral reconstitution of the tibial-peroneal trunk more distally (*arrows*). This case represents another complication of popliteal aneurysm, namely spontaneous thrombosis. Since there is often a poorly developed collateral network in these patients, severe ischemia is common when thrombosis occurs.

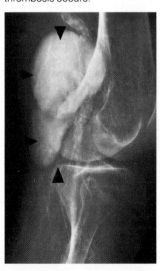

Fig. 5.7 An uncommon complication of popliteal aneurysm is spontaneous rupture. This patient presented with an acutely enlarging mass behind the knee as well as severe ischemia in the lower leg and foot. This late-phase film from a femoral arteriogram demonstrates filling of the popliteal bursa with contrast (*arrows*), representing free rupture of the aneurysm.

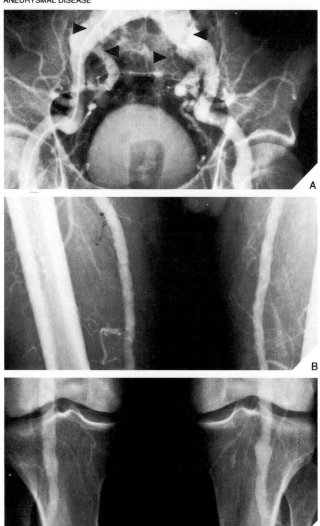

Fig. 5.8 Arteriomegaly is a generalized vascular disorder manifested by diffuse widening of the blood vessels as well as frank aneurysm formation. **A, B, C** Three films from a peripheral arteriogram in a patient who was originally being studied for an abdominal aortic aneurysm demonstrate arteriomegaly. Note the aneuryms of the common iliac arteries. (**A**, *arrows*), with diffuse widening in all of the distal vessels. It is likely that popliteal aneurysms are actually present and contain laminated thrombus, preventing visualization of the entire aneurysm sac.

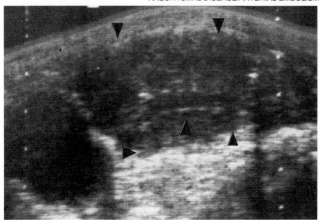

Fig. 5.9 An ultrasound study of the popliteal region was necessary to confirm the presence of an aneurysm. Note the echo-free central lumen (*arrow* 1) and the surrounding thrombus (*arrows* 2).

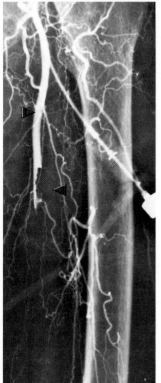

Fig. 5.10 A 62-year-old woman with a long history of atrial fibrillation was admitted with acute ischemia of the left leg from the thigh to the foot. This film of the thigh from a femoral arteriogram demonstrates no visualization of the superficial femoral artery, a finding that could be acute or chronic in nature. The deep femoral artery (*arrow* 1) is occluded in the upper thigh and there is a sharply marginated, lucent filling defect just above the point of occlusion (*arrow* 2). This intraluminal filling defect is the key to making the diagnosis of embolus. Other suggestive findings include the abrupt cutoff of the vessel and the relative lack of collateralization distally. Given the history of atrial fibrillation, this embolus is most likely of cardiac origin.

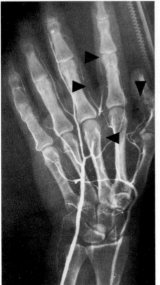

Fig. 5.11 Small emboli frequently lodge in the most distal segments of the circulation, often manifested clinically by isolated ischemic fingers or toes. A 52-year-old woman was noted to have several blue, painful fingers a few days after subclavian artery surgery. The arteriogram demonstrates numerous distal occlusions (*arrows* 1). A filling defect can actually be seen within a metacarpal vessel (*arrow* 2), confirming the embolic nature of the problem.

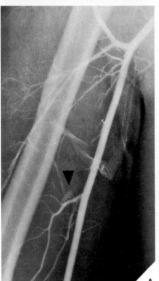
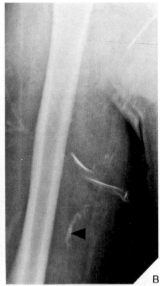

Fig. 5.12 **A** This patient fell through a plate glass window and on admission was found to be bleeding heavily from the upper arm. The arteriogram demonstrates an irregular collection of contrast next to one of the brachial artery branches (*arrow*). **B** The late-phase film demonstrates persistence of the contrast collection in the same region (*arrow*). These findings are typical for extravasation.

88

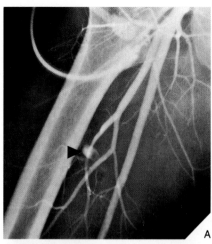

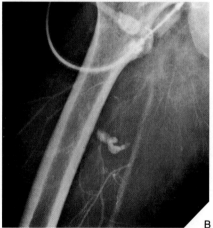

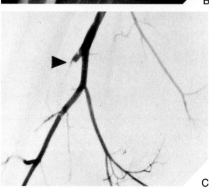

Fig. 5.13 A A patient suffered a stab wound to the inner aspect of the thigh. At that time a hematoma was noted but there was no evidence of continued bleeding. He was admitted one month later with an enlarging mass in the thigh following heavy exertion. The arteriogram demonstrates a pseudoaneurysm from a branch of the deep femoral artery (*arrow*). B The late-phase film shows stasis of the contrast within the pseudoaneurysm. It must be appreciated that the pseudoaneurysm is generally surrounded by a much larger hematoma than would be indicated by the opacified sac. C Transcatheter embolization was performed using stainless steel coils, resulting in occlusion of the traumatized branch (*arrow*) and control of the hemorrhage without the need for surgery.

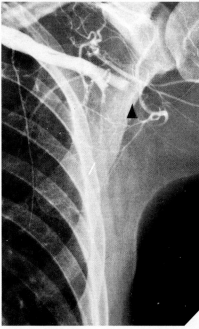

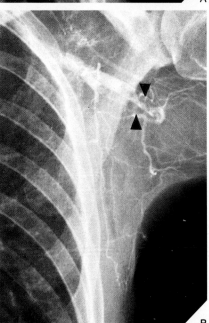

Fig. 5.14 A
Occasionally,
vascular trauma is
caused by a less
obvious inciting
factor. For example,
this patient
developed acute pain
in the left upper
extremity after
attempting to push a
heavy object. The
arteriogram
demonstates abrupt
occlusion of the
midportion of the
axillary artery (*arrow*).
B The late-phase film
demonstrates fresh
thrombus within the
vessel (*arrows*) and
stasis of contrast.
This type of
thrombosis is
presumed to be
caused by extrinsic
muscular trauma to
the vessel.
Angiographically, this
would not be
distinguishable from
a large embolus in the
axillary artery.

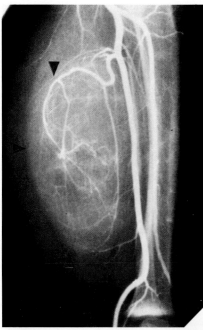

Fig. 5.15 **A** An eight-month-old child was found to have a firm mass in the calf on physical examination. The arteriogram demonstrates a hypervascular mass supplied predominantly by branches of the posterior tibial artery (*arrows*). **B** Dense staining is noted on the late-phase film. Surgery revealed a soft tissue sarcoma.

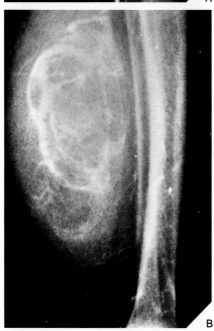

91

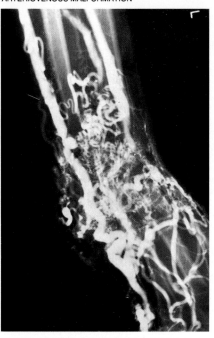

Fig. 5.16 This 49-year-old man had an arteriovenous malformation of the left arm and hand since childhood. Amputation of two fingers and a portion of the palm of the hand was performed in separate procedures. The arteriogram at this time demonstrates extensive residual malformation involving the remaining fingers, the palm, and the distal forearm. Note the marked enlargement of the radial and ulnar arteries (*arrows*), typical of vessels supplying a high-flow lesion.

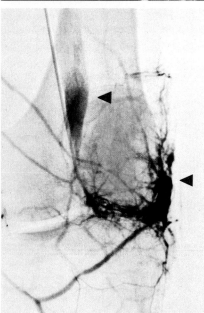

Fig. 5.17 An 18-year-old man had a subtler type of arteriovenous malformation that caused pain in the lateral aspect of the knee. The catheter was selectively placed in one of the small geniculate branches. Numerous abnormal arteries are visible (*arrow* 1) and there is shunting into the popliteal vein (*arrow* 2). This lesion was successfully treated by embolization through the catheter and no surgery was required.

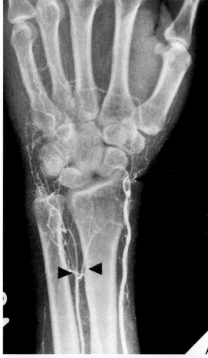

Fig. 5.18 **A** This hand arteriogram of a 59-year-old man with nonspecific vasculitis demonstrates abrupt narrowing of the radial, ulnar, and interosseus arteries in the distal forearm (*arrows*). The vessels of the palm and digits show marked irregularity as well as segmental occlusions. **B** The magnification study of the fingers demonstrates these findings more dramatically (*arrows*). The diffuse nature of the problem and the irregularity of the vessels rule out emboli as a diagnosis, and atherosclerosis rarely involves the upper extremity in this way.

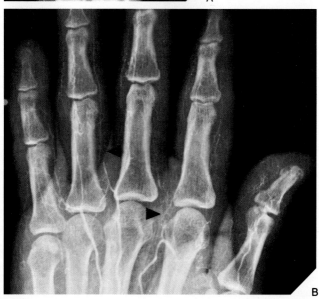

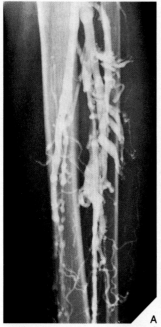

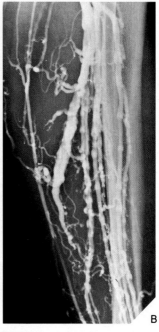

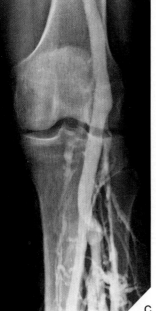

Fig. 5.19 A, B, C, The anatomy of the venous system in the lower extremities varies much more than the corresponding arterial anatomy. This study of a normal leg demonstrates that the multiplicity of superimposed calf veins may make it difficult to exclude the presence of deep venous thrombosis. Therefore, oblique views are generally taken of this region. Interpretation is simpler at the popliteal and higher levels. Generally, the deep venous system up to at least the external iliac level can be visualized during venography.

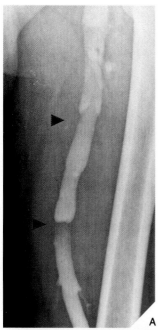

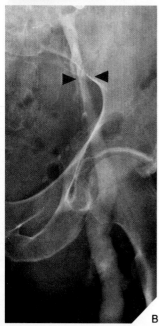

Fig. 5.20 A, B Note the appearance of normal venous valves in the femoral vein of the thigh (**A**, *arrows*). There is slight extrinsic narrowing of the iliac vein in this case due to a pelvic mass (**B**, *arrows*).

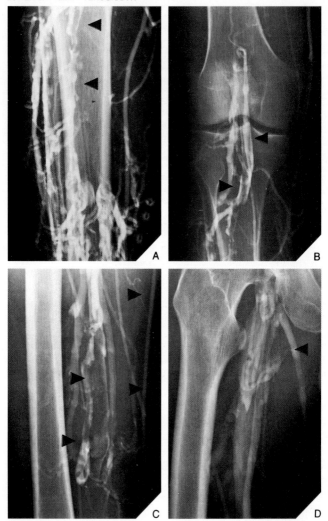

Fig. 5.21 A, B, C, D This venogram sequence of the right leg demonstrates the typical findings of acute deep venous thrombosis extending from the calf veins to the common femoral level. To make a firm diagnosis, acute thrombus must be visualized within the deep veins as seen here in the upper calf, popliteal region, and thigh (*arrows* 1). A small amount of contrast generally flows around the thrombus, producing a ghostlike appearance. Nonfilling of deep veins may suggest the diagnosis of DVT; however, this finding is not in itself sufficient to make a diagnosis. Note the normal saphenous vein in the medial soft tissues, a part of the superficial venous system (*arrows* 2).

96

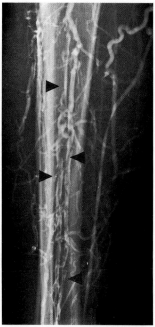

Fig. 5.22 This is another example of extensive deep venous thrombosis involving the calf veins. Note that almost every deep vein contains an elongated lucent filling defect representing thrombus with contrast passing around it (*arrows*).

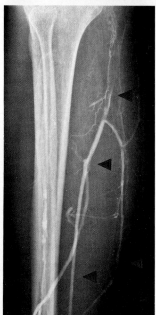

Fig. 5.23 In some cases, the deep veins may be so completely filled with thrombus that essentially all of the venous flow is diverted into the superficial veins (*arrows* 1). In this case, some clot material is also present in the superficial veins (*arrow* 2). Generally at least one segment of the deep vessels can be seen with thrombus in the lumen. If repeated attempts show no filling of the deep system, a diagnosis of complete thrombosis can be made.

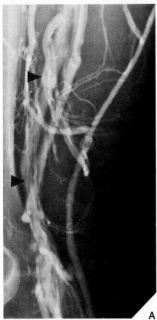

Fig. 5.24 A, B When deep venous thrombosis is adequately treated and has clinically resolved, there usually are no abnormalities visible on follow-up venograms. Occasionally, recanalization of the thrombi will be incomplete and fibrin strands will persist in the lumen of the veins. This development produces a "webbed" appearance consisting of fine linear defects or striations, as seen here in the veins of the popliteal and thigh region (*arrows*). Webbing may be associated with extensive destruction of the venous valve system and subsequent venous valvular insufficiency. Sometimes the webbing is so extensive that it is impossible to completely rule out the presence of a superimposed acute thrombosis.

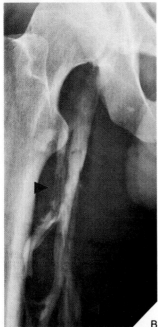

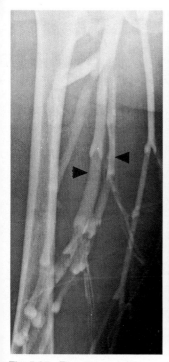

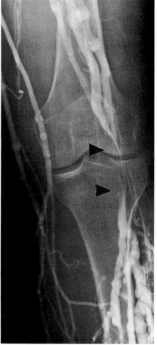

Fig. 5.25 The anatomy of the peripheral venous system is highly variable, a fact that one must constantly bear in mind when interpreting leg venograms. In this case there is a double femoral vein (*arrows*) in the thigh. While this is of no significance in itself, the diagnosis of DVT could be missed if one femoral vein thrombosed while the other remained patent.

Fig. 5.26 Any extrinsic mass can cause displacement and compression of the normal veins in the extremity. If the compression is severe enough, it may actually result in a secondary thrombosis below the site of obstruction due to stasis. In this case, there is a marked extrinsic compression of the popliteal vein almost to the point of complete occlusion (*arrows*). The smooth tapered nature of the defect as well as the lateral displacement indicate that this is an extrinsic problem rather than intrinsic venous disease. The differential diagnosis would include soft tissue tumor, a large popliteal aneurysm, or, the correct diagnosis in this case, a large Baker's cyst. An ultrasound study of this region confirmed the presence of a cystic mass and a normal popliteal artery.

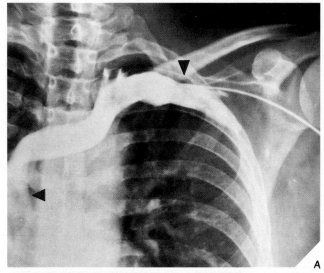

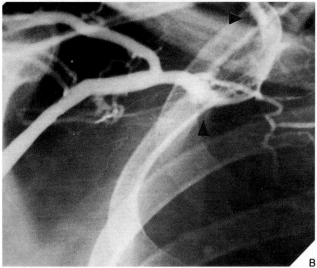

Fig. 5.27 **A** This is a normal subclavian venogram performed by inserting a catheter through an antecubital vein and passing it proximally into the distal subclavian vein. The study demonstrates a widely patent subclavian vein (*arrow* 1) draining into the superior vena cava (*arrow* 2). **B** This film demonstrates the typical findings in subclavian vein thrombosis with complete occlusion of the subclavian vein (*arrow* 1) and filling of collateral venous pathways (*arrow* 2). The collaterals typically drain through the jugular circulation and less commonly through the chest wall.

6
Lymphangiography

Diagnostic Usage and Usefulness (Figs. 6.1–6.4)

Lymphangiography, a rather involved procedure for visualizing the lymph nodes in the abdomen and pelvis, is usually employed in the diagnostic work-up of malignant disease, especially pelvic tumors and lymphomas. With the advent of computed tomography (CT) and ultrasound, which can demonstrate the presence or absence of gross lymph node enlargement, lymphangiography is performed much less often. However, when the CT scan is equivocal or normal, a lymphangiogram may be helpful in showing subtle abnormalities, such as filling defects or changes in texture, that could indicate the presence of malignant disease.

The study involves a minor surgical procedure, to permit direct exposure and cannulation of the lymphatic channels on the dorsum of each foot and slow injection of an oily iodinated contrast medium. Films of the abdomen and pelvis are obtained immediately after completion of the injection in what is called the channel phase; another set of films is taken 24 hours later, in the nodal phase, when contrast has left the lymphatic channels and lodged in the pelvic and para-aortic nodes. The contrast remains in these nodes for several months and can be seen on plain radiographs.

Normal lymph nodes vary markedly in appearance but tend to have an elongated bean shape and a dense granular texture. They are intimately associated with the iliac arteries, and longitudinal grooves may normally be seen in the pelvic nodes, representing vascular impressions.

Malignant involvement of the lymph nodes may result in nodal enlargement, changes in the internal texture (e.g., the "foamy" nodes seen in lymphoma), sharply marginated filling defects (usually associated with metastatic disease), or complete replacement of the node by tumor. The latter may result in a complete lack of opacification, but the diagnosis can sometimes be suggested by obstruction of lymph channels with persistent filling of dilated channels on the nodal-phase films, which are normally free of contrast by that time.

Lymphangiography is also performed occasionally to investigate suspected non-malignant lymphatic problems, such as congenital abnormalities, unexplained edema, or involvement of the lymphatic system by trauma.

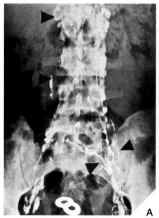

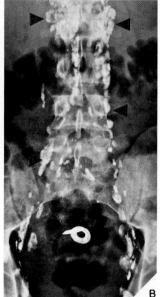

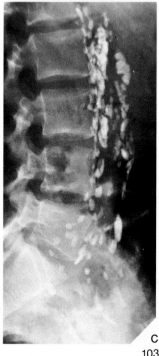

Fig. 6.1 In a study performed as part of the diagnostic evaluation of a 19-year-old man with known Hodgkin's disease in the mediastinum, these normal lymphangiograms were obtained. **A** A channel-phase film obtained immediately following contrast injection through the lymphatics in both feet clearly demonstrates the lymphatic channels (*arrows* 1), as well as early filling of the iliac and para-aortic lymph nodes (*arrows* 2). Little diagnostic information is usually available in channel-phase films except for the suggestion of obstructed or displaced channels. **B** On a nodal-phase film, obtained 24 hours after injection, there is good opacification of the iliac and para-aortic nodes (*arrows* 1). Note the normal elongated bean shape of the lymph nodes with their homogenous yet somewhat granular consistency. When many lymph nodes are superimposed on each other (*arrows* 2), one can appreciate the difficulty in ruling out a filling defect. **C** Lateral, as shown here, and oblique films can usually separate the nodes enough to determine the presence of defects.

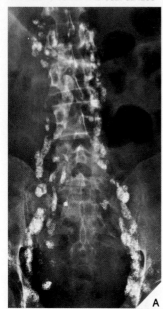

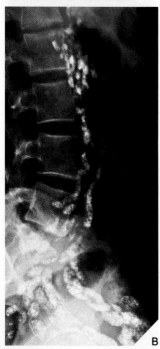

Fig. 6.2 A, B Positive nodal-phase lymphangiogram of a 35-year-old man with known Hodgkins's disease demonstrates enlargement of all of the iliac and para-aortic nodes. More important is the alteration in the normal texture of the nodes, with numerous small filling defects and a generalized "foamy" appearance. These findings are typical of lymphomatous involvement, confirmed in this case at laparotomy.

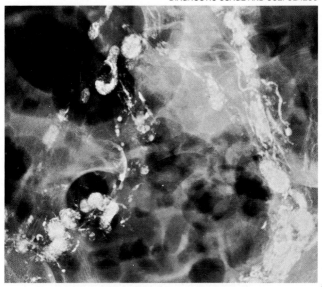

Fig. 6.3 Positive lymphangiogram in a patient with metastatic cervical carcinoma demonstrates a sharply marginated filling defect (*arrow*) suggestive of metastatic disease. There is considerable variation in the lymphangiographic appearance of lymphoma and metastatic disease; the two are not always distinguishable.

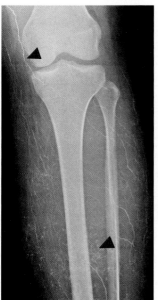

Fig. 6.4 In a 20-year-old woman being evaluated for unexplained edema of the left leg, venograms (not shown) were negative. This channel-phase lymphangiogram demonstrates the fine caliber of normal lymphatic vessels in the extremities (*arrow* 1). The irregular collections of contrast material scattered through the soft tissues (*arrows* 2) are consistent with dermal backflow generally encountered in lymphatic obstruction. In this case severe inflammatory disease caused obstructive changes in the pelvic nodes on this side.

General References

Abrams HL (editor): Angiography, 3rd ed. Little, Brown, Boston, Massachusetts, 1983.

Athanasoulis CA, Pfister RC, Greene RE, Roberson GH (editors): Interventional Radiology. WB Saunders, Philadelphia, Pennsylvania, 1982.

Kadir S: Diagnostic Angiography. WB Saunders, Philadelphia, Pennsylvania, 1986.

Neiman HL, Yao JST (editors): Angiography of Vascular Disease. Churchill Livingstone, New York, New York, 1985.

Index